RESEARCH METH
HEALTH SCIENCES

RESEARCH METHODS FOR THE HEALTH SCIENCES

D.A. Brodie
J.G. Williams
R.G. Owens*

Department of Movement Science and Physical Education,
The University of Liverpool

and

*Health Studies Research Division
University of Wales, Bangor

harwood academic publishers

Australia • Canada • China • France • Germany • India • Japan • Luxembourg • Malaysia • The Netherlands • Russia • Singapore • Switzerland • Thailand • United Kingdom

First published 1994
Second printing 1997

 Printed in Singapore.

Amsteldijk 166
1st Floor
1079 LH Amsterdam
The Netherlands

British Library Cataloguing in Publication Data

Brodie, David A.
Research methods for the health sciences/D.A. Brodie.
J.G. Williams, R.G. Owens.
p. cm.
Includes bibliographical references and index.
ISBN 3-7186-5527-6
1. Medical sciences – Research – Methodology. 2. Allied health personnel. I. Williams, J.G. II. Owens, R. Glynn.
III. Title.
R850.B76 1994
610′.72-dc20 94-1258
CIP

CONTENTS

ACKNOWLEDGEMENT

We wish to record our thanks to Debi Leonard, secretary in the Department of Movement Science and Physical Education at the University of Liverpool, for her commitment to the task of converting our initial drafts into camera-ready copy and for her patience in tolerating numerous revisions.

PREFACE

This book is designed to provide an introduction to research methods for students from the Health Science subjects of physical education, sports studies, movement science, nursing, physiotherapy, occupational therapy, clinical psychology, public health and the imaging sciences.

The book is to be used primarily for undergraduate students in the above sub-disciplines, but it is considered that many postgraduates who have not had a good grounding in research methods will also find the book useful.

The many practical examples throughout the book will be deliberately chosen to illustrate the principles and practice using simple experimental equipment which is either commonly available or could be produced cheaply and easily. This has two advantages:

(i) the book could become a lecture course because the practical work is an inherent part of the learning process, and

(ii) students can work independently and follow up the lecture sessions with home-based practicals.

It is designed to enable a student to:

Understand what is meant by research, and to appreciate the breadth of activities subsumed under the term;

Convert general and possibly ill-specified questions into hypotheses appropriate for scientific investigation;

Understand the variety of ways in which researchers gather their data, the advantages and disadvantages of the various methods, and the way in which the methods relate to the topics and questions of interest;

Conduct simple group experiments and simple quasi-experiments and to analyze the results obtained using basic statistical procedure;

Conduct simple small-N experiments using a range of designs;

Conduct simple pieces of ethnographic research, and perform basic analyses on the data obtained;

Provide appropriate interpretations of the data obtained from each of the various response styles;

Understand the principle whereby the simple experiments performed may be converted into more sophisticated forms using refinements of the procedure;

Prepare a written account of research projects in a form suitable for publication within the scientific literature;

Evaluate critically existing published studies, treating such reports with an appropriate degree of caution;

Know how to extend the knowledge derived from the book itself by further reading and involvement in practical exercises.

The book is structured in three parts. The first provides the general conceptual principles necessary for an application of research methodologies. The second part illustrates practical application of these general principles, showing the reader how to conduct particular forms of research and indicating how results obtained may be analyzed and interpreted. For each of these areas instructions are given on how to perform basic analyses. Also provided is an outline of the principles underlying more complex procedures when detailed discussion is beyond the scope of the book.

To enliven the text we have included wherever possible specific examples of research techniques from the various sub disciplines of human movement and health sciences. These include examples from exercise physiology, biomechanics, clinical psychology, physiotherapy, nursing and others. These are normally incorporated in the case studies but reference to applied research techniques are also within the text.

The third section returns to an important aspect of research, criticism and dissemination. It is intended to give specific guidance which should enhance the standard of work in terms of research output.

Each individual chapter is tightly structured to give clarity and consistency throughout the book. Each chapter contains:

1. Key words
2. Introduction
3. Main text
4. Exercise and/or review questions
5. Summary
6. References (when applicable)

Within some chapters the reader will note some text in an unnumbered box. This will relate to material which can be read independently from the general text.

The appendices provide additional information which will be of value to the reader.

PART I: *RESEARCH PRINCIPLES*

The first two chapters in this book introduce the reader to the topic of research and set out principles which are an essential foundation to the skills of the researcher. Chapter 1 deals with definitions and concepts concerning the research process. Chapter 2 provides a frame of reference and explanations of the strategies used by researchers to elicit facts which is the main purpose of research activity.

Each chapter comprises a section on the issues, exercises, and a summary. The exercises are designed to establish a conceptual framework for Part II which is about Research Practice. Research skills are acquired through 'doing after planning' rather than by way of reflective processes. The exercises should be useful in thinking things through carefully before acting. Some works and terms are highlighted (italicised). These relate to important concepts so should be accorded particular attention.

CHAPTER 1

THE RESEARCH PROCESS

Key words : *problem; literature review; evaluation; proposition; fact.*

What Is Research?

Research is about obtaining the facts concerning a particular phenomenon or problem. In a sense most adults and even children spend a portion of each day, perhaps unwittingly, involved in research in order to conduct their lives in an equable fashion. Virtually everyone has to acquire factual information to enable them to make decisions. This process forms the basis of the way humans behave and how the world works. The popular conception of research is that it is work done in a laboratory, but the workplace, home, school, and library are all legitimate foci for fact-finding activity. Indeed such places can become research 'laboratories' themselves.

A moment's reflection can provide numerous instances of research activity and illustrate some important principles. For example, today I am in a foreign country and have to travel from one town to another in order to keep an appointment. The distance to be travelled is some 200 kilometres and I possess the resources (skills and funds) to make the journey. I have never been to where I am going and possess very little knowledge of where I am at the present time. Prior knowledge of keeping appointments myself and the behaviour of others who have done similar activities informs me that I shall have to move from point A (present location) to point B (desired location) within a given time. In the current circumstances such information is too general to be of practical use. I must obtain some facts which will help me get myself to where I want to be or find someone who knows the way and is willing to take me. In short, I have a *problem* and must do some research if I am to make my appointment on time.

Problems And Solutions...

The word ‘problem’ is well known in everyday language and is also a key term in the language of the researcher. The first task in a research project is to define the problem concisely. In the example, the problem is pretty straightforward. It has been clearly stated that I have an appointment in a given place at a given time and need some facts on how to make the journey from my present location. Although my current knowledge of the geography of the two places is scant, I do know that there are various utilities for getting me to where I wish to go. Research should provide an answer to my problem!

If it were the case that the purpose of my research was to produce a useful, generalizable guideline on travelling to keep appointments in foreign countries then it is highly improbable that such an objective could be achieved economically. The process of clearly defining the problem is seldom easy but absolutely essential and must be considered to be a prime tenet of successful research. A useful first step in delineating the problem is to pose this question. Is there a potential solution to the problem? Only if the answer is positive is it likely that a tenable problem can be formulated.

To return to the example, the problem is clearly formulated and a solution probable. The burning question is how will research help me to attain my objective? One option open to me in travelling to keep my appointment is just to set out. I try to convince myself that I can gather information and make the necessary decisions along the way. Before electing this option I pause to consider my first decisions and the consequences of making an error. Which mode of transport do I use? Which way to I go? I soon realize that I shall need a ‘plan’ for reaching my destination and the better the information contained in the plan the less frustrating and time wasting my journey will be. This situation illustrates a further research principle, namely, the requirement for a *plan of action* that will result in arriving at an acceptable solution to the problem.

Plans And Existing Information...

When considering the available options for getting to my destination on time, it soon became clear to me that a planned approach to the problem would probably be preferable to a trial and error approach. Of course, there may be occasions when the latter is the only available option and may have to be used whilst implementing a given plan of action.

One of the surest aspects of human problem solving is that others have been confronted with similar situations. Often their experiences and solutions for given problems will be documented or stored in either written or experiential form. The facts may have been disseminated quite widely. The individual or group who has tackled a given problem may be available for advice or consultation. This is an important resource for the researcher. Finding out about the experiences of others and evaluating these is another important principle in research which features early in the formulation of a plan for addressing a problem. This part of the process is usually referred to as *'reviewing the literature'*.

In the case of my travel-to-appointment problems there is a great deal of human experience of this to the extent that my research will consist of first finding out more about where I am and where I want to go. Secondly I need to establish the travel facilities available to transport me to my appointment on time. In common with other researchers I am faced with the task of tracking down the sources of the information that I require.

The next stage in my problem brings forth a further research principle. With the necessary facts before me I am placed in the position of having to *evaluate* the information and decide which mode of conveyance will get me to my appointment on time. Walking and cycling are both too slow so I have to develop a *proposition* or *prediction* (often referred to as a hypothesis) from the available facts whether I should go by train, bus or motor car. Because this was a 'one-off' appointment, time did not permit me to obtain the travel time information for the various travel options by experiencing them for myself and then deciding which was best (empirical approach). It was necessary to make the decision from the findings of others, namely, train or bus schedule times or estimates of motoring times and distances. Nonetheless, it was necessary for me to assess the probability of timely arrival and predict which would be the most efficient way of travelling to my appointment.

Researchers evaluate the information that they have collected to produce what they believe to be facts. The end products of the research process are to set out the facts and to predict the probability of event occurrence from them.

As a matter of interest, I purchased a map, hired a car, formulated a strategy and used this, with a small amount of trial-and-error, to solve my problem! I now possess facts concerning that particular problem gathered from direct experience, albeit a single instance, for arriving at a satisfactory solution. The research process, systematic acquisition of the facts, facilitated a satisfactory answer to the problem.

Exercise 1.1

Select a 'problem' from your own area of interest in the same manner as the 'travel-to-appointment' example used to explain the key features of the research process in this chapter. Use pencil, paper and eraser (or word processor with cut and paste facility!) to set out a plan for both obtaining and presenting the facts for the given problem and the steps you would take to ensure that the information is accurate. Quite a good idea is to develop a 'flow chart' comprising the various phases and stages that you would go through from the point at which the problem was concisely defined to the point when the facts are presented.

Exercise 1.2

Explain by writing in your own words the meaning of the following terms:

> Research, problem, prediction, proposition, hypothesis, review of literature, evaluate, fact, truth, probability.

Summary...

This brief introduction has defined research using an everyday example to introduce several key features of the research process. The points made can be summarized as follows:

1. Research is about obtaining the facts pertaining to a particular problem.
2. Research methods and techniques can be applied to virtually any problem and are not limited to the popular image of the laboratory and white coat.
3. In order to obtain the facts, a particular problem has to be defined precisely and a solution a realistic probability.
4. Sound research emanates from well laid plans showing how the necessary facts will be obtained. Although trial and error strategy is sometimes unavoidable, the planned, systematic approach is preferable.
5. An important aspect of problem formulation and planning is to determine as thoroughly as possible what others have found in the given or directly related area.
6. Researchers evaluate the information that they have gathered to determine the extent to which the information is 'true' and, sometimes, predict the probability of occurrence of given events from the facts in their possession.
7. Finally, researchers report the findings of their studies and 'bank' the facts in such a way as to make the details available to others who may have an interest in the problem. In this way a contribution to the store of knowledge for a given area is augmented and developed.

CHAPTER 2

STRATEGIES FOR OBTAINING FACTS

Key words : *control; retrospective; prospective; experimental; inferences; dependent; independent; internal validity; external validity.*

It has been established that research is concerned with obtaining the facts for a given problem. As stated above, researchers seek the 'truth'. However, because of uncertainty concerning the accuracy of the facts which contribute to the truth, they have to arrive at decisions which reflect the *probability* of things being true. The major difficulty faced by the researcher's quest for the facts relates to the degree of *control* exerted over the events that generate information connected with the problem. The greater the control, the higher the probability that the facts will be accurate and representative of the truth.

There are many different types of research and various strategies for attempting to ensure the accuracy of the findings. Rather than categorize the numerous varieties of research, the approach here is to characterize research activity by developing the notion of *control*. This refers to purposeful procedures used by a researcher to minimize the amount of error in the data collected. Error is an inherent element of all information. In a fact-finding activity it has to be minimized so that alternative explanations for given findings are limited and generalization beyond a particular instance is possible.

Researchers seek to attain a high level of *validity* (truthfulness) by ensuring that any measurements taken, measure what they purport to measure and that error is not unwittingly introduced into the data collection process by way of procedural anomalies. An example from an area of public health research is used here to introduce various classes of research and typical control problems which have to be addressed by the research worker.

During the past twenty or so years there has been a great deal of interest among health researchers in coming to understand the cause of coronary artery disease (CAD). CAD has an extremely high incidence in industrialised societies such as the USA and Western Europe. The disease is a major cause of death and disability. Because CAD can take thirty to forty years to manifest itself, early research was faced with the considerable problem of looking back into such records as were available in an attempt to determine the antecedent factors which ultimately result in large numbers of people becoming ill or dying. Looking at past records to establish why things happened is perhaps the most common method of doing research. Here, this method will be referred to as 'retrospective'.

The Retrospective Approach

A typical retrospective strategy would be to first propose some phenomena likely to be associated with the symptoms of the illness, then carry out an analysis of the relationship between the criterion phenomenon (CAD) and the phenomenon(a) thought to be responsible (say incidence of smoking, level of total blood cholesterol etc) and report positive/negative association. In 'retrospective' or 'what happened' research, the investigator has very little control over the quality of the data which is necessary for arriving at a tenable answer to the problem. The available data collection strategies are mainly limited to the acquisition and interpretation of health records which may not be in a form that is pertinent to the research problem. Frequently, interviews are conducted or questionnaires completed. These methods of data collection depend heavily on the respondents' memories for an accurate representation of events.

Plainly, the conscientious researcher wishing to gain knowledge of the causes of CAD would be unhappy with limitations imposed by having to look back over considerable periods of time and having to interpret records which were registered by others and not necessarily of direct relevance to the problem in question. A researcher undertaking studies of this kind is faced with severe control problems because there is little that can be done to ensure the accuracy of the available data. Nevertheless, whilst this approach is not in itself definitive it can serve the purpose of offering 'leads' to some of the key factors associated with a research problem. Thus, a retrospective approach is a tenable method of doing research and may be the only strategy possible for a given problem but it does not permit levels of control when collecting and interpreting data that a researcher would really like to exert. This said, there are some advanced analytical techniques designed to minimize errorful conclusions being drawn which are applied routinely in this area but these are beyond the scope of the present text.

The Prospective Approach

In order to counteract the shortcomings of the numerous retrospective studies in research into the causes of coronary artery disease there was clearly a call for much improved control over the data collection process. It was suggested that the validity of the findings would be improved by adopting a *'prospective'* or 'will it happen' approach. Rather than attempting to make sense of events that have already happened, this strategy tries carefully to monitor events as they occur. This is done by, first, delineating the variables (phenomena) believed to be associated with the development of CAD such as high blood pressure, lack of exercise, stressful occupational circumstances etc. Then, after carrying out assessments at regular intervals in a representative sample of a given population over a lengthy time period, reporting any associations between the predictor variables and the eventual development of the disease.

The research strategy described is widely used in the study of epidemics (epidemiology). There are a number of now famous prospective studies aiming to monitor and report on variables which are believed to be related to the development of coronary artery disease. The Framingham Study which has been systematically monitoring the onset and development of CAD within an entire community near Boston in the United States of America is a prime example of the prospective approach and has been running for some twenty years. The results are reported regularly in the *American Journal of Epidemiology*.

There is little doubt that a prospective approach to a research problem permits the investigator to exert greater control over the data collection process than the retrospective approach. Recall that in the latter, the investigator was forced to interpret existing data rather than ensure that appropriate measurements were taken then transform data of known validity into information. This is a distinction of great importance in research and is one aspect of the very essence of *control*.

Despite the improvements in control offered by the use of a prospective research strategy in the efforts to understand the causes of a complex phenomenon such as coronary artery disease, a moment of reflection will reveal to the reader that there remain numerous variables which still present the researcher withserious control problems. Items which spring readily to mind are 'human' variables such as changes which might occur in a person's behaviour from being part of a study especially when the topic concerns health and well-being. In short, a prospective strategy enables a researcher to plan ahead, decide which subjects will be studied, use measurement devices of predetermined quality and, within reason, monitor events as they are happening. As good as this sounds, as ever, there are a number of detractors which are especially prevalent when the subjects of the research are human. Even with the best laid plans and efficient research design, the multifaceted nature of people and their various activities introduces control problems for the researcher. Humans are mobile, have widely differing genetic make-up, varied personality, many physical characteristics, malleable attitudes and motives, and are sensitive to social pressures. These factors and others create special problems in acquiring facts about them. This difficulty is particularly acute when attempting to solve a puzzle such as the causes of coronary artery disease which is almost certainly a function of a complex interaction of numerous variables over a lengthy span of time.

The Experimental Approach

Given the shortcomings of both the 'retrospective' and 'prospective' approaches for the CAD example begs the question, "is there a strategy which ensures the level of control necessary for obtaining the facts?" The answer is a conditional 'yes'. What might be termed the "gold standard" strategy is probably the model of control that researchers would like to emulate if the nature of their particular problem permits this to be applied. This is commonly referred to as the *experimental method*.

Ideally researchers prefer to observe events directly, as they are happening. For example, if I proposed that regular vigorous exercise exerted a beneficial effect on individuals with the symptoms of coronary artery disease, I should ideally want to see for myself the flow of blood within the arterial system and just how the diseased organs were affected. Of course, ethical, technical and economic constraints limit my capacity to do this so most research is a compromise. This results in the application of the *best methods for the particular problem*.

The unique circumstances of experimental method are that the researcher is prepared for observation, makes events occur, varies conditions systematically while noting any variations in the results and, under some conditions, repeats observations to verify the result. When these circumstances are attainable the degree of control exerted by the researcher is closer to optimal and it is expected that the probability of obtaining accurate information is very high. In essence, the experimental method represents a standard of control *to be* achieved rather then a standard which *is* achieved especially in human research. This is due, in part, to the fact that the origins of experimental design and statistical analysis lie in horticulture research. It is self-evident that the application of the experimental method with plants as subjects is somewhat easier than controlling human variability!

Research into aetiology (causes) of coronary artery disease provides examples of the quest for better control in the attempt to obtain the facts. At the same time it illustrates the reality of applying experimental method with human subjects in the context of a complex problem. Here it will be used to demonstrate the researchers' control strategies and prime considerations in presenting the facts and establishing cause and effect relationship. An experimental approach would be required to provide direct anatomical evidence of the effects of given doses of exercise on the coronary arteries as opposed to implied evidence.

A general hypothesis could be that exercise protects against coronary artery disease. A typical research hypothesis would propose that *if* people (referred to as 'subjects') engaged in regular vigorous exercise, *then* fewer signs of CHD, for example, as indicated by coronary artery diameter would be evident. With the problem defined and a hypothesis stated it is possible to track various facets which are-searcher takes into account prior to collecting data and drawing conclusions concerning causality. In the present example, this would be that regular exercise maintains the diameter of the coronary artery and thereby allows adequate blood flow to the heart muscle.

The essence of experimental method is that it offers a strategy for investigating the effects of one or more *variables* on one or more other variables while controlling for (ruling out) the effects of other factors in order to draw *valid inferences* (facts or probably truth). The variables of direct interest to the experimenter are normally referred to as *dependent* (sometimes called 'criterion' or 'performance') and *independent* (sometimes called 'predictor'). These should be self-evident in the hypothesis.

In the example, level of CAD (dependent variable:diameter of coronary artery) is a function of vigorous exercise (independent variable). The researcher designs the experiment so as to minimize the effects of other variables so that unambiguous inferences can be drawn from the results of the experiment. The prime goal of the researcher is to implement a valid plan with the twin purpose of ruling out rival hypotheses or alternative explanations (*internal validity*) and being able to generalize the findings beyond the unique circumstances of the experiment (*external validity*).

Researchers usually refer to 'threats' to validity. The main detractors from the attainment of validity (those other than the independent variables of specific interest in the experiment) are explained below under the appropriate subheadings.

Internal Validity

The 'history' of the subject and significant events occurring during the research project such as personal problems and crises can influence results. Also, maturational changes resulting from adaptations within a person e.g. ageing, becoming healthier, getting fitter etc. Change which originates from repeated exposure to testing is another potential source of error which could lead to false conclusions. In a similar vein, changes may occur in measurement devices or assessment procedures during the course of a research project. These may be human or instrument adaptations (or a combination of both) and can distort results. Extreme values, say for scores in an assessment procedure, tend to revert toward the average of scores for a given group (an effect termed statistical regression) and may change the direction of scores from one assessment to another. Bias in initial subject selection and loss of subjects during a project can lead to observed differences between groups which reflect differences in these events rather than any effect brought about by an independent variable. Finally, diffusion of treatment including subtle alterations in the effects of an independent variable which can occur as an experiment proceeds (e.g. differential use of praise or encouragement while administering a procedure) is another factor which can lead to false conclusions being drawn.

External Validity

Validity is compromised if there are doubts as to whether the results of research can be extended across subject, settings, tasks and time-of-day. Furthermore, subjects' behaviour and performance in research investigations can be influenced by their awareness of being singled out for a particular treatment, being assessed or sensitized to the effects of a particular treatment before it occurs. If the research examines the effects of a number of levels of an independent variable upon a dependent variable, interference which limits the generality of the result may occur. For example, the results may apply only to others who are treated in the same way or same order.

Clearly, the process of *control*, as potential threats to validity in an attempt to rule out alternative explanations and generalize results, is far from being a trivial matter. A researcher has to achieve a balance in controlling threats to external and internal validity; unnecessary severity or negligence on either side will result in distortion of the facts.

Exercise 2.1

Go back to the hypothesis which was advanced for examining the effects of exercise on coronary artery disease then consider the following questions carefully:

1. Is there a potential solution to this problem?
2. Can this hypothesis be tested?
3. Could an experimental approach be applied?
4. Could human subjects be used?
5. Define the dependent variable. Can it be measured accurately and consistently?
6. Consider the independent variable(s). How would the effects of this (these) be administered?
7. Carefully re-read the sections on internal and external validity. Spend some time considering variables that pose a threat to validity and the steps that would be taken to control these in an experiment.

When this has been done the reality of experimental method as the standard for approaching research in a *controlled* manner and, thereby, minimising error becomes apparent. This exercise is a useful preparation for the next chapter.

Summary

1. Researchers attempt to obtain the facts and ascertain the probability of finding out what is true *(valid)*.

2. All information contains an element of error which detracts from the quality of the facts. Researchers go to great lengths to minimize error by doing their best to *control* the data collection process. Sound information on a problem could be conceived as comprising 'facts' and 'artefacts', the latter being the error.

3. The precise nature of the problem and the circumstances of a particular project dictate the researcher's approach to securing the facts. Broadly speaking an attempt is made either to interpret events that have already happened (*retrospective* approach) or to investigate events as they occur from a given point in time (*prospective* strategy).

4. A 'model' strategy is the *experimental* method. With this approach the researcher hypothesizes a casual relationship between a given *dependent* variable and one or more *independent* variables at the same time *controlling* for other variables which could permit alternative explanation of the findings and limit their generalization beyond the particular circumstances of the experiment.

5. The strength of the experimental approach lies in the potentially high level of control exerted in the fact gathering process whereby the researcher has planned ahead and is ready for observation, makes events occur, and systematically varies conditions noting any alterations in the results.

PART II: *RESEARCH PRACTICE*

Whereas the first part of this book advanced some important principles and general strategies of research, this section introduces the reader to the various ways of actually doing research. When one considers the profusion of phenomena about which humans would like to acquire facts, it is unsurprising that a wide range of techniques for obtaining and interpreting information have been developed and others are still developing. Research in the human movement and health sciences is well versed in using such techniques in the process of acquiring knowledge. What follows is a representative sample of how researchers in this field tackle various tasks. The purpose is to provide a conceptual framework on how things are done as a basis for thought, decision-making and reflection about individual research problems and potential solutions. Fine details and definitive answers to each and every research question are not provided. Important terms and ideas are highlighted (italicized) and should be given special attention.

CHAPTER 3

EXPERIMENTS

Key words : *random; population; pseudo-experimental; quasi-experimental; law of parsimony; design; mixed; order; standardization; F-ratio; critical value; interaction; post-hoc tests.*

The purpose of this chapter is to explain the process of setting up and running experiments then interpreting the results and drawing conclusions for a given hypothesis. The explanation will be illustrated by use of a contrived but realistic and comprehensive example which describes and elaborates on the emergence of a research problem. It shows how a plan for systematic acquisition of the facts can be developed and conclusions drawn from careful observations made under controlled conditions. This process is commonly referred to under the global term *experimental* design.

Before entering into the details of this chapter it is important to emphasise that the reader should focus on developing a sound understanding of the principles of experimental design concentrating upon the notion of *control* introduced earlier. It is vital that the processes for obtaining factual information relating to a particular problem are thoroughly understood. The reason for making this statement is that experimentation is essentially a two-part, integrated process comprising methods for collecting data with respect to the hypothesis (research plan) and the use of 'tools' for interpreting the data (statistical analysis). Although a sound working knowledge of both elements is essential for doing quality research, many people who would like to do research become excessively concerned in grappling with the fine details of statistics in the first instance. It is preferable to invest effort into grasping the concepts initially, then, to spend time learning to use the wide range of items which are available in the statistical 'toolkit'. Nowadays, there are many user-friendly, 'expert-system' statistical analysis packages for use with microcomputers which considerably reduce the effort involved in the 'arithmetic' tasks. The reader is urged to concentrate on *why* particular statistical manipulations are carried out to help make decisions for given hypotheses. The emphasis in the analytical sections of this chapter is on the meaning of a particular approach rather than mathematical formulae and computation.

Types Of Experimental Study

The term 'experimental' requires clarification. The content of this chapter addresses what are termed 'true' experiments. In these the researcher is able to fulfil all of the criteria necessary for carrying out an experimental study. Recall from the previous chapter that for optimal control the researcher is organised and prepared for observation, makes events occur and varies conditions noting any fluctuations in the results. Sometimes observations may be repeated (replicated) in order to verify findings. In addition to these procedural constraints the subjects in a study will have been *randomly* chosen from *the population at large* and their treatment under the independent variable will be compared to results obtained by accepted strategies of experimental control.

The entry criteria for 'true' experiments are stringent. Frequently, a research problem does not permit one or more of the necessary standards to be met. In these circumstances the researcher may adopt an experimental approach in a study but must be prepared to defend criticisms concerning the validity of any conclusions drawn. These designs are referred to as '*pseudo*-experimental' and '*quasi*-experimental'.

The descriptor pseudo (false) applies to any design in which there is a critical absence of control. Studies in which this occurs are far more prevalent in the research literature than might be expected. Most readers will be familiar with the classic example. The formal name is the "one-group, pretest-posttest design". With this design the researcher first tests subjects on a given performance variable say, level of physical fitness, then administers a treatment which is predicted to significantly influence fitness level (a vigorous exercise programme). Following this, fitness level is assessed again and conclusions drawn as to the effects of the treatment by comparing the subjects' performance on the pretest with that on the posttest.

The reader should think back, or refer again, to the sections on research design validity in the previous chapter and consider carefully which uncontrolled variables could be confounded with the effects of the independent variable (the exercise programme) in the above example. You will probably be able to detect as many as five (history, maturation, instrumentation, statistical regression, and attrition). It is worth remembering that these extra variables become rival hypotheses to the prediction that physical fitness level is significantly influenced by involvement in a given exercise programme.

The message for the novice researcher is loud and clear. When adopting an experimental research strategy think the design through very carefully so as to avoid the descriptor 'pseudo' by considering the potential threats to research design validity and, as far as possible, *controlling* them. If your design acquires the pseudo label you will never convince people that conclusions drawn concerning your hypotheses are factual.

Experimental research becomes 'quasi' (almost) experimental when the nature of the study does not permit certain control procedures to be adopted. For example, the researcher may not be able to dictate when observations can be made or where and when an independent variable is manipulated with a given group of subjects. Quasi-experimental designs are common in health and human science research. For example, it could be predicted that in certain stroke patients, the ability to grasp objects is improved when treated using visual feedback from the action-potentials of the finger muscles. It is clear from the outset that, although the researcher might proceed with an experimental ethic, the criteria for true experimental method are unlikely to be attained.

Once again, readers should recall the categories of threat to the validity of a study and consider the influence of doing research in an 'almost' experimental manner. As a general rule, it will be concluded that true experimental designs can have greater control over internal threats to validity and quasi-experimental designs can have greater control over external threats. As ever, most human endeavour requires compromise. The conscientious researcher strives to achieve control as much as possible, so as to maximize the chance of obtaining facts.

Example Of An Experiment

Already, it will be clear that the main purpose of an experiment is to test a hypothesis or make predictions by controlling as many variables as possible except those that are the focus of interest in the hypothesis. As one might expect, experimental designs will vary in complexity depending on the nature of the problem being studied and the number of predictions the researcher is attempting to make.

An important tenet of experimental research is referred to as the *law of parsimony*. This states that "entities should not be replicated without necessity". This in practice, means that the researcher should derive as much information as possible without waste of time and effort. This can be achieved by resourceful experimental design.

One way of doing research (and learning about research design) would be to begin with an apparently simple plan which compares the effects of two conditions (levels of an independent variable) on a dependent variable. For example, examining the effects of step aerobic exercise versus conventional aerobic exercise (two levels of an independent variable) upon physical fitness level (one level of a dependent variable). Some reflection on this approach would likely draw comments of the "how about a, b, c?" variety or "how will you account for x, y, z"; queries which dispute the validity of the design because certain important factors will not be accounted for or *controlled*. In short, this type of plan is simple to execute but not easy to defend. In reality, very few research problems can be reduced to a straightforward comparison of the effects of two experimental conditions. The outcome has been that students of research methods have confronted this predicament and have evolved experimental plans of action which both control and maximize the amount of information for hypothesis testing. Such designs are commonly referred to as 'complex'. Perhaps a more appropriate term would be 'comprehensive' because these are merely more detailed versions of the instance referred to above as simple. The example to be worked through now is comprehensive in nature but not complex.

Problem

A person in the field of 'Active Health' develops an intuition while teaching exercise classes that the physical exercise itself exerts the effect of altering the mental alertness as well as physical fitness in the participants. Toward the end and just after the exercise classes people seem to be more attentive, observant, and responsive in their actions. If this 'hunch' were confirmed by sound research some claim could be made for positive psychological as well as physiological effects to exercise.

This possible bonus leads the individual to try to establish whether any evidence exists for this proposition. Library research reveals some plausible speculation that exercise could alter brain biochemistry in such a way that a person would become more vigilant and attentive. Also, that some empirical research had been undertaken on this topic for which the findings were equivocal; some supporting the proposition, others reporting null results. These studies had been criticised on the grounds of inadequate design and lack of consideration of certain potentially important variables connected with the exercise treatment effect.

The active health practitioner decided to examine the proposition by carrying out an experiment designed to rectify, as far as possible, the shortcomings which had been indicated in previous research. This should adequately test the general hypothesis that physical exercise will significantly influence mental awareness.

Design And Method

The researcher has access to a relatively large group (approx. 500) of healthy, moderately fit young adults (aged 22–25 years) who participate regularly, twice per week, in aerobic-type physical activity and is able to specify comparable maximal aerobic capacity and intellectual capability. It should be noted that this group constitutes a 'convenience' sample rather than one which has been randomly drawn from the exercising population at large thus limiting external validity.

Design Decisions

The researcher considers the group which comprises both men and women and the potential effects of exercise on mental functioning and reasons that the process would probably be uninfluenced by gender. Although it is known that men and women approach exercise tasks in a different manner which might affect the outcome, the generally recreational nature of this type of exercise would probably not produce gender specific results. So, a mixed gender group of eighty subjects is randomly drawn from the larger group. This number is based on considerations of the time, cost and general practicalities of the testing procedure set against the number of observations which is mathematically necessary for a 'fair' test of the hypothesis. In reality, some thirty subjects per condition would be preferable to satisfy the latter condition.

Before proceeding, the ethics of experimentation requires that the researcher obtains individual, written informed consent for each subjects participation in the experiment. This is acquired while making every effort to minimize their sensitivity to the precise details of the hypothesis which is to be tested and so avoid influencing the validity of the study.

The next decision to be made concerns a design criticism arising from prior research on this topic. A critical review of previous research suggests that various facets of the independent variable, exercise, had not been carefully considered. For example, most people who have been involved with physical exercise understand the significance of specifying important dimensions of activity such as 'intensity' (how hard will it be?) and 'duration' (how long will it last?). Both factors either individually or in combination could affect mental alertness one way or the other. Similarly, there is the question of when a change in mental alertness, if any, will take place. Would there be an immediate effect on alertness? Is it possible that any effect would be delayed until a point when some recovery had been made from the exertion? Would any positive or negative effect be transient or would it last? Furthermore, the researcher might ponder whether any effects brought about by the exercise might not be constant but vary with the level of another variable. Such an effect is referred to as an *interaction*. For example, an improvement in mental alertness might be evident following exercise *but only* when the exercise was of a given intensity *and only* if the activity were of given relative duration. That is to say that a person may have to work pretty hard before a noticeable change occurs but if they work hard for too long any positive alteration in alertness may be impaired, perhaps by fatigue.

Within reasonable limits resourceful experimental design includes logically important factors in the plan rather than eliminating them. So a comprehensive design should have the outcome of generating more information and controlling elements that are likely to influence the hypothesis.

In theory, virtually any number of variables and levels of variables could be incorporated into a design. In practice, unnecessary inclusion is also unparsimonious. In the present example, *two* levels of each of *two* independent variables, namely, 'relative exercise intensity' (light and hard exercise) and 'relative exercise duration' (short and long exercise bout) are examined. For the sake of example, mental alertness, is measured at an individually judged point in the post-exercise period.

Same Or Different Subject?

A further consideration in designing an experiment which involves exposing subjects to different independent variables is whether to use the *same* subjects for each of the different conditions, or *different* subjects for each of the variables. Such designs are commonly referred to as related or unrelated respectively (sometimes as correlated/uncorrelated or within/between). Sometimes the experimenter uses the same subjects for some variables and different subjects for the others. This is referred to as a *mixed* design.

Plainly, there are advantages in being able to use the same subjects for each of the conditions in the experiment but some obvious disadvantages too. Perhaps the strongest reason is that the researcher can minimize the effect of unwanted individual differences which may affect subjects' response to the experimental tasks. Level of motivation for being involved in the experiment, for example, would be about equal for all conditions. However, the disadvantages lie in factors such as fatigue inherent in the tasks, sensitization of subjects to the purpose of the experiment, and the possible influence of carrying out the experimental conditions in a particular *order*. The experimenter has to weigh up the pros and cons, with the criterion of design validity foremost in mind.

In the present example, the researcher is as sure as possible about the homogeneity of the group with respect to some potentially crucial individual differences and is concerned about both sensitization (exposure to the mental alertness assessment) and the confounding effects of fatigue because of the intensity and duration of certain exercise conditions. The decision is made to use a between-subjects design (different subjects in each of the experimental conditions).

Measuring The Dependent Variable

The researcher must use a valid and reliable measure of the dependent (performance) variable. It has been hypothesized that physical exercise increases mental alertness. Plainly, 'alertness' could be conceptualised in a number of ways. Here it is taken to be 'vigilant' and 'attentive' as measured by the time it takes an individual to process a visual signal and execute an accurate movement response (reaction time plus movement time). For the sake of the example, the researcher is able to test subjects on a computerized driving stimulation task in which it is possible to programme the brake lights of a vehicle ahead to come on at random intervals and accurately record braking response time by the driver of the following vehicle; alertness is taken to be a function of speed of response. This is a sophisticated version of some contemporary computer games.

Also the researcher is able to introduce subjects to this task and verify that their performances fall within the normal range for adults. The sample was judged to be comparable in physical fitness, psychomotor performance, general intellect, and biographical variables. The performance variable measure is a specially derived interval scale score ranging from 1-slowest to 4/5-average to 9-fastest computed from the raw response time values from ten trials at the mental alertness task.

Specifying The Treatment Variables And Running The Experiment

The researcher has prior knowledge of the physical activity of the subjects, e.g. how often they exercise, the duration of their exercise session, and their fitness level. Confirmation that their reaction times and movement response times are within the 'normal' range is available. The question remains as to which exercise duration, exercise intensity and periods of recovery should be selected as treatments to examine the effects of exercise on mental alertness.

The researcher decides on cycling (familiar activities to the subjects) on a cycle ergometer which permits the duration and intensity of exercise relative to each subjects' fitness level to be accurately assessed and administered. The two intensity levels of the cycling exercise selected are 55% (low) and 75% (high) of individually estimated maximal capacity and verbally reported by all subjects to feel 'light' and 'hard' respectively during test trials to develop the experimental procedures. The duration levels are set at 10 minutes (short) and 20 minutes (long) taken from the subjects' collective perception of a relatively brief or extended bout of exercise undertaken in the early evening. Relative recovery time is set individually by monitoring each subjects' heart rates and taken to be 50% of the highest heart rate in beats per minute observed during the exercise bout.

Next, the researcher has to work out a procedure for what is referred to as *'running'* the experiment. That is to say the manner in which the subjects will be exposed to the treatment or experimental variables so that the effects of these on the dependent or performance variable(s) can be realistically assessed. The implementation of the procedure must be meticulous because this process is a potential source of error in itself. The researcher *standardizes* the circumstances for receiving the subjects, preparing them for involvement in the experiment, giving instructions for what they have to do, ensuring that their participation in the experiment is optimal, collecting performance data, and reinstating all subjects to their pre-experimental level. The experimenter makes every effort to ensure that his or her actions conform with accepted ethical standards for the participation of human subjects in research studies. The researcher may either practise the procedure for running the experiment to iron out any snags or difficulties in the procedure or train a suitable person to administer the protocol to avoid possible experimenter bias.

Finally, subjects are randomly allocated to experimental conditions by a person other than the researcher. Then, an appointment schedule is arranged for each subjects' involvement in the experiment. The experiment is 'run', data collected and analyzed.

In summary, the researcher has designed an experiment to test the hypothesis that "aerobic exercise of given intensity and duration will cause a positive and significant alteration in mental alertness at a specified point in the recovery period following large muscle group physical activity". A sample of adult subjects of similar age and general background, fitness level and psychomotor ability were randomly allocated to four experimental conditions (two levels of exercise intensity times two levels of exercise duration) which culminate in a test of mental alertness. The researcher uses a statistical technique called multivariate analysis of variance (MANOVA) to determine the effects of the independent variables (intensity and duration) on the dependent variable (mental alertness) *and* any interaction effects. The results permit statements to be made about the hypothesis. The performance scores on the mental alertness test for each subject in each condition of the experiment are submitted for computer analysis. Contemporary statistical analysis packages provide the results in seconds. The researcher's task is to interpret the results and draw conclusions.

Results

The underlying principle of the statistical technique which has been termed MANOVA is that it is a method of calculating quantities of variance due to all possible sources of variability in the subject's performance scores. All tests of human subjects will yield variation in score value. Some of this variation will be due to *true* differences between individuals (or groups which comprise individuals), the remainder will be due to error in the measurement process. The researcher's goal is to minimize *(control)* the error portion and maximize the true portion. MANOVA is a method of parcelling the *total variance* in performance under the experimental conditions into *true* variance and *error* variance. The relationship between these two classes of variance is expressed as a ratio. This is referred to as the *F-ratio.* The numerical value of the F-ratio is frequently referred to as the *critical value* because it alone summarizes the outcome of the analysis. The smaller the error portion relative to the true portion, the larger the F-ratio and the more confident the researcher can be that the effects of an independent variable are 'real' rather than due to chance or error. Conversely, the larger the error variance relative to the true variance, the lower will be the F-ratio and subsequently the researcher's confidence that observed differences are factual ones.

The results of the MANOVA are normally set out in a table for ease of interpretation. Table 3.1 below provides the results of the present experiment set out in the way it would look from a computer printout. In the first column

Table 3.1: Typical computer printout for a MANOVA

	Summary of all effects; design:					
Error	df Effect	MS Effect	df Error	MS Error	F	p-level
*1	1	4.05000	76	.425000	9.5294	.002822
*2	1	57.80000	76	.425000	136.000	.000000
*12	1	84.05000	76	.425000	197.7647	.000000

* Marked effects significant at p<.0500

(labelled 'Effect') are set down the effects of the independent variables and the interaction between the variables. In the third column (labelled "MS Effect") the numbers represent the 'true' variance for the independent variables and in the fifth column the 'error' variance within the variables. Columns two and four mention 'df' or degrees of freedom. The faith that can be placed in the accuracy of statistics is very much a function of the size of the sample of observations taken. This point was made earlier in the example when the sample size and number of subjects per condition was stated. Degrees of freedom are always one (1) less than the total number of observations. So in column two, the number 1 is one less than the two levels of each independent variable whereas in column four, the number (76) is arrived at by multiplying the number of conditions (4) by one less than the number of subjects in each of those conditions (19). The sixth column (headed 'F') refers to the F-ratio arrived at from the ratio of column three ('true' variance) and column five ('error' variance). The last column on the right of the table provides the probability level for the F-ratio value. The asterisks in the first column indicate probabilities of the calculated F-ratio regarded as significant. That is to say that this value would occur by chance on 5% or less occasions. The significance level of the F-ratio is confirmed by checking it in a table of probabilities which are normally positioned in the appendices of statistical texts (contemporary computer packages such as used in the present analysis provide significance levels). Many researchers believe that if a critical value (F-ratio) is significant at the 5% probability level that some degree of faith can be placed in that result. This is a philosophical issue in research. It is sufficient to say here that the 5% level of significance is frequently considered to be a relatively tangible boundary for distinguishing 'fact' from 'fiction'!

When scanning the MANOVA table it is evident that the first two of the experimental conditions (intensity and duration), taken alone, significantly altered mental alertness in some way. However, the striking aspect of the experiment is the *interaction*. Recall that an interaction occurs when the level of a variable is not constant but changes with the level of another variable. In the present example it certainly seems to have been a prudent decision to use an experimental design that permitted these effects to be demonstrated.

Probably the soundest way to understand the effects of one variable on another is to consider the mean response time standard scores in each combination of conditions and then examine these pictorially. Table 3.2 shows the mean values (remember that the standards range from 1-slowest, through 4-5 average, to 9-fast). Figure 3.1 is a graph of the interactions in which the line plots represent the levels of intensity (high-continuous line and low-broken line) and duration (long and short) set on the horizontal axis. Response time is on the vertical axis.

Table 3.2: Mean values for the response timer

		MEANS
INT	DUR	RT
HIGH	LONG	3.500000
HIGH	SHORT	7.250000
LOW	LONG	5.100000
LOW	SHORT	4.750000

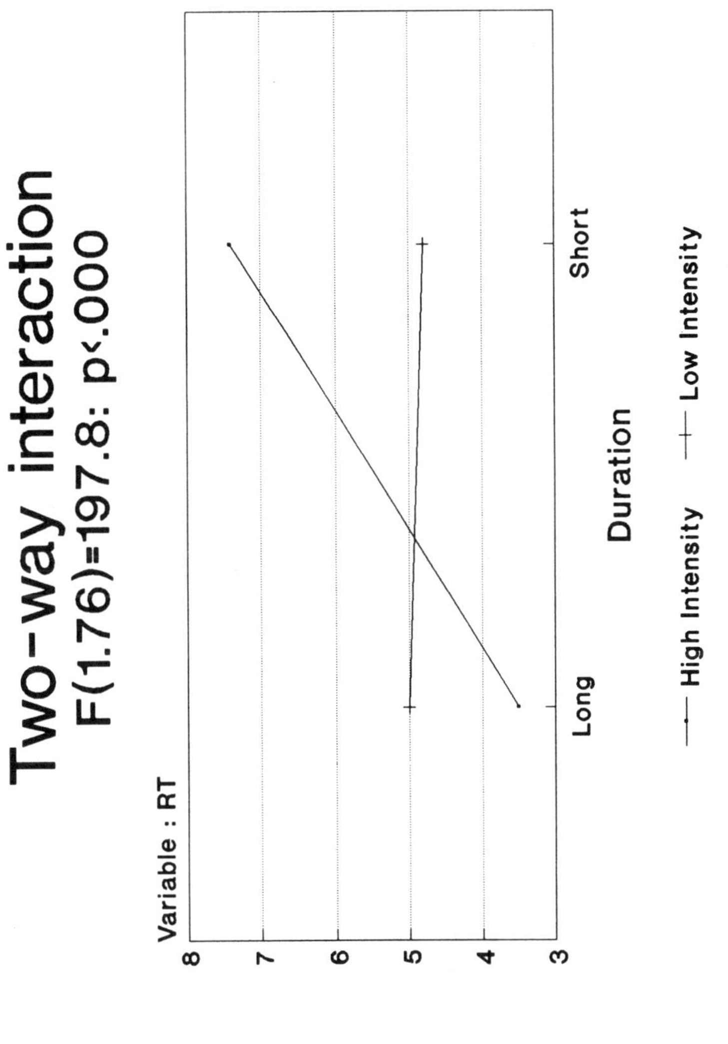

Figure 3.1: Graph of the interactions between duration and intensity

Table 3.3: Probabilities for the Tukey *post-hoc* test

		Tukey LSD test; variable RT Probabilities for Post-Hoc Tests INTERACTION: 1 × 2			
		(1)	(2)	(3)	(4)
INT	DUR	3.500000	7.250000	5.100000	4.750000
HIGH	LONG (1)		.000148	.000148	.000148
HIGH	SHORT(2)	.000148		.000148	.000148
LOW	LONG (3)	.000148	.000148		.332091
LOW	SHORT(4)	.000148	.000148	.332091	

It is clear that the low intensity bout of cycling exercise produced similar, about average reaction times irrespective of whether it was of long or short duration. However, the intense cycling exercise had a very different effect. A long-intense bout apparently blunted alertness. Conversely, a short duration bout of high intensity exercise resulted in a dramatic quickening of mental alertness.

Graphing the interactions serves to clarify the effects but does not confirm them. Pictures can be misleading! Thus, the researcher carries out a series of follow-up statistical tests in order to specify, precisely, any differences between the conditions. These mathematical manoeuvres are known as *post-hoc* tests and are usually available as an option with a statistical analysis package. There are numerous versions of follow-up tests and a full explanation of decisions and choice related to these is beyond the scope of the present text. Suffice to say that the test used here has been accepted by statisticians as reliable for making such comparisons.

Briefly stated, post-hoc tests make pairwise comparisons of mean values whilst maintaining the pre-established level of significance (taken to be pi.05 in the present example). Table 3.3 provides probabilities for the Tukey test which was applied in pairwise fashion to the mean response time scores computed for the six pairs of mean scores in the example experiment. These results can be interpreted by referring back to the graph of the two-way interactions. Once again this table shows how results come off the computer. Taking the blanks in the table as a diagonal line, it is only necessary to consider one or other side of this diagonal as results to either side of the diagonal are mirror images.

For the most part, the graph portrays an accurate representation of events. There were no significant differences in mental alertness following either long duration or short duration low intensity exercise ($p=0.332$). However, all other differences were significant ($p<0.002$). Plainly, the high intensity dimension of the exercise exerted the most potent effect on mental alertness as measured by response time.

Given the circumstances of the experiment, the active health researcher's initial hunch that exercise rendered people more mentally alert was conditionally confirmed by the results of controlled experimentation. That is to say that a short duration, high intensity bout of cycling significantly increased mental alertness, as defined in this experiment. Also, by taking account of a number of exercise-related factors within a comprehensive research design, quite a lot of additional information was gleaned. Not least that under certain conditions there was either no notable effect at all or, in the case of a physically demanding dose, what could be considered a detrimental influence in that it slowed down mental alertness substantially.

The researcher would write a comprehensive and concise report of the finds and conclusions of the experiment and submit these to the editorial panel of a journal in the relevant field (see Chapter 10). The conduct of the research would be reviewed by experienced researchers in the area. If considered fit for publication, the paper would subsequently appear in the journal to be read and considered by other active health practitioners as part of the knowledge-base of workers in the field. The experimental results should contribute to the various dimensions of the role of exercise as a part of a healthy lifestyle.

Exercise 3.1

Look back over this chapter focusing in particular on the example which was offered. Re-examine the manner in which the hypothesis evolved, the plan was formulated, the independent variables and the dependent variable were defined. Consolidate how the experimental procedure was worked out, how the experiment was run and the data acquired and interpreted. Attempt to ensure that you understand each of these phases and the reasons why things were done. Discuss the methods with other students or individuals who have done some research. Think through and note any limitations in terms of internal and external threats to validity. In doing this focus not so much on the subject of the experimental example but on the methods and the results upon which conclusions were drawn.

Now take a pencil and paper and address each of these stages with a fresh problem. This could be completely contrived or a 'real' problem of interest that you would like to solve. Write down a working hypothesis and, then, express a more precise hypothesis or prediction. Delineate several independent variables and levels of these variables. Define the performance variable, how it will be measured and what the units of measurement will be. Work out and write down a design and procedure for exposing the subjects to experimental treatments.

Exercise 3.2

Prepare a sample record sheet which specifies each of the conditions and record some imaginary scores (say ten observations per condition) then derive average scores both in line with your prediction and against your prediction. Plot the score on an interaction-type graph as given in Figure 3.1 of the example and spend some time working out what the results mean.

Exercise 3.3

Finally, rough out a short report with an introduction to the problem, a precise purpose for the experiment stating the hypothesis. Next write out the design of the experiment with the dependent measure, then specify the procedure that the subjects went through. Finally, attempt an interpretation of the results in relation to your hypothesis using the mean values and the graph.

If you have not taken a course of formal instruction in research design and statistical analysis but have acquired a reasonably sound understanding of this and the previous chapters you should have no qualms about undertaking such a task. If you have undertaken an introductory course and experienced some difficulty, these first chapters should serve to clarify the necessary concepts for this topic.

Summary

1. Experimental studies often include choosing subjects at random, but other designs (e.g. quasi-experimental) are also used. This will occur when controls are less stringent.
2. As many variables as possible should be controlled except the variable(s) of interest.
3. It is necessary to make a number of design decisions based on availability of numbers, ethics, and prior research.
4. It is essential to decide whether the same or different subjects will be studies as part of the experimental design. Experimental order also has to be considered.
5. The statistical method of calculating the quantities of variance due to all possible sources of variability in the subjects' scores is the MANOVA. It is important to establish the interaction.
6. *Post-hoc* tests examine the pairwise differences between mean values.

CHAPTER 4

WHAT'S THE DIFFERENCE?

Key words : *null hypothesis; alternative hypothesis; mean; sample; unbiased; median; mode; type I and type II errors; population; mean deviation; variance; standard deviation; t-statistic; degrees of freedom; significant; one-tailed and two-tailed tests; nonparametric.*

Chapter 3 gave a review of the process of experimentation and used as illustration a fictitious design from active health. This chapter consolidates certain experimental features introduced earlier and does so by examining a common research problem — do differences really exist between groups?

Let us imagine that a practice nurse in a doctor's surgery has decided to undertake total blood cholesterol screening as part of a 'well woman' clinic. She is able to borrow a reflotron dry chemistry analyzer to see whether it would be appropriate for her use. She recalls that total blood cholesterol tends to be higher in older people so decides to examine two different groups of subjects (patients), one old and one young. We are now aware of biological variability and numerous other variables which could influence cholesterol apart from age, but for the purposes of this study let us assume that they are at least recognized, if not controlled.

It is now worth re-stating what the practice nurse wishes to examine. Remember our suggestion in Chapter 2 that hypotheses can be written as *if....then....* statements.

Exercise 4.1

Write the research problem under discussion as *if....then....* statement before turning over the page to see our solution.

If age is a factor in total blood cholesterol *then* the nurse should observe clear differences between the results from the older and younger groups.

Your hypothesis was unlikely to be identical to this but you will know if you are close. Health and human scientists tend to state hypotheses in a slightly more formal style and adopt what is called a *null hypothesis*.

In the present example, the null hypothesis (H_0) is that "there is *no* difference between the two groups" and that any difference between them is simply a result of chance variation. It is like the differences we would have obtained if we had simply taken successive individuals, whether old or young, as they entered the well woman clinic.

Some researchers re-state the hypothesis as an *alternative* (or experimental) *hypothesis (or* H_1*)* and this simply states that "there is a difference between the two groups."

Exercise 4.2

Write out a series of null hypotheses and alternative hypotheses related to the general hypothesis that physical exercise will significantly influence mental alertness. If you have difficulty return to Chapter 3 and review what was initially done.

Write out some null hypotheses for a hypothetical experiment involving two groups from your own area of interest. Start each one with H_o=.....

The following table gives the results from the two groups, rounded off to the nearest mmol l^{-1} for reasons of simplicity.

Table 4.1 Hypothetical cholesterol data from 20 subjects.

Group 1 (*Young*)		Group 2 (*Old*)	
Subject No.	Cholesterol (mmol l^{-1})	Subject No.	Cholesterol (mmol l^{-1})
1	2	11	6
2	3	12	8
3	5	13	7
4	4	14	5
5	3	15	4
6	4	16	8
7	6	17	9
8	4	18	7
9	5	19	6
10	4	20	5

How do we decide whether or not there is really a difference between the two groups? Looking at the data the second group do seem, in general, to contain higher values than the first group. However this isn't always the case, and some of the subjects in Group 1 (e.g. subjects 3, 7 and 9) have higher scores than the lowest (subject 15) in Group 2. Clearly then the subjects in the second group do not *always* score higher than the subjects in the first group. This is not so surprising; most of the time when we compare one group with another we obtain a certain degree of overlap; what we are interested in is not so much whether *everyone* in one group scores higher than another, but rather whether one group *tends in general* to score higher than another.

An obvious course of action is to compare, not the individual scores, but instead the means or average scores for the two groups. A quick calculation will show that Group 1 has a mean score of 4.0 and Group 2 a mean score of 6.5. We might be inclined to conclude that the second group do tend to have higher scores than the first. Before rushing to such a conclusion, however, it is worth thinking a little more deeply. Mean scores of 4.0 and 6.5 are indeed different, but considering the fact that the individuals within the groups vary among themselves, and that we only have ten people in each group, we probably would not expect the two groups to have *exactly* the same mean score.

Central Measures

The *mean* is another name for the 'average' you learned at school, obtained by adding all the individual scores and dividing by the total number of observations. This can be summarised by the equation $\sum x/N$ where x refers to each individual score, $\sum x$ means add each individual score together, and N refers to the total number of observations (in our example, ten in each sample). The mean of a *sample* like this can be used to estimate the mean of the population from which it the sample has been drawn. Indeed the sample mean is sometimes referred to as an *unbiased* estimator of the population mean.

The term 'mean' is used in preference to 'average' because statistics recognized several kinds of average including the *median* (obtained by listing the observations in order and taking the middle value, or for even-numbered samples the mean of the two middle values) and the *mode* (obtained by determining which is the most common value in the sample). Try to determine the median and mode for the twenty numbers in Table 1 (you should obtain values of 5 and 4 respectively).

You should also note that, strictly, the *mean* referred to here should be called the *arithmetic mean*; there are other types of mean such as the geometric and harmonic means, which are used in particular circumstances.

So how much of a difference do we look for between the two samples before concluding that they do indeed represent a real difference? If the two groups had means of 4.0 and 5.5 would we be persuaded? Suppose they were 4.0 and 4.5? Or 4.0 and 4.1? Probably if you ask around you will find that people differ as to how much of a difference they would want to see before being persuaded that there was a 'real' difference between the groups. Clearly what we need here is a rather more objective basis for deciding how much of a difference we need to see before being persuaded.

A moment's reflection will reveal that there are actually four possibilities; either there is or there is not a difference between the two groups, and we can be right or wrong in drawing our own conclusion on this question. Table 4.2 illustrates the possibilities;

Table 4.2 The ways in which we might be right or wrong

There really is a difference, and we draw the correct conclusion.	There really *isn't* a difference but we mistakenly conclude that there *is* (a *Type I* error).
There really *is* a difference but we mistakenly conclude that there *isn't* (a *Type II* error).	There really isn't a difference and we draw the correct conclusion.

The distinction between types of error made in Table 4.2 is important. It is generally felt that in science it is more serious to make a Type I error than a Type II error. Every time a new variable is introduced into a scientific study a considerable amount of effort is expended into determining exactly the form of the relationship, under what circumstances it holds etc. If in the end it was found that there was no such relationship after all, the effort would have been wasted. As a result statistics have given itself an intentional bias, such that the chances of a Type I error are deliberately kept below a certain level. A large number of statistical procedures have now been devised which mean that, under certain circumstances, we can conclude that two (or more) variables are related knowing that as long as we use these procedures we will only be wrong fairly infrequently.

We still have to decide whether or not the two means we have obtained (4.0 and 6.5) are sufficiently different for us to be justified in concluding that the two groups really do differ? Our null hypothesis is that the difference we have obtained is simply due to chance variation. If chance were *indeed* the only factor operating, would we be likely to obtain a result like the one above?

At first glance this might seem like an impossible question to answer. How can we know how often a result like this would arise by chance? We do have a clue. If we look at out figures, we realise that besides sampling the actual scores it also samples the variability of the scores. The extent to which the individuals in our samples vary gives us an indication of how much variation we might expect in the wider populations from which they have been sampled. The detailed mathematics of doing so needn't concern us; formulae for doing this have been derived by others and used as a basis for devising statistical tests to deal with particular experimental questions. These methods enable us to take samples of data and by applying the appropriate formulae to calculate how likely our results would be to occur simply by chance. Thus, in effect, a statistical test of our present data would calculate the mean difference between the two groups, calculate the variability between the individuals, and on the basis of these tell us how likely such a result would arise by chance. If such a result was extremely *unlikely* the only remaining hypothesis is that there is a *reason* for the difference, i.e. that the two groups really *do* differ with respect to the characteristic in question.

Measuring The Variability In Our Data

If we want to know how likely our results are to occur by chance, one thing we need to know is how much variability there is in the data. If data do not vary at all — if every individual scores the same — then a sample can only end up with that particular value as the mean. For example, if everyone obtains a score of five, then no matter how many samples we take, all of them will have a mean of five. On the other hand if our data vary, then there are more possibilities for the mean to take. It is important to be able to obtain some kind of measure of variability in our data, if only to use this as an estimate of the amount of variability in the population from which our sample has been drawn.

Samples and Populations

The terms 'sample' and 'population' are used in a specific way in statistics. A sample is a set of individuals who are felt to be representative of some large group or population. Thus there can be many types of population; the population of students, of marathon runners, of male sprinters, of female high jumpers etc. Samples may be drawn from any such group and used to draw inferences about the wider population in question.

In fact there are a number of ways of measuring variability. Most rest on the idea of calculating how much the data in a sample vary around the mean. Thus in a sample of numbers like 4, 5, 4, 5, 4, 5, 4, 5 we have a mean of 4.5 (do the calculation to check, if you like) and each number is 0.5 away from the mean. Thus the *mean deviation* of the sample from the mean is 0.5 — that is to say, on average each number is 0.5 away from the mean.

A more common estimate is the *mean squared* deviation. In this the mean is calculated, then each number is subtracted from the mean, and the result is squared. Each of these squared numbers (there are as many as there were original numbers in the sample) is then added together and divided by the sample size (usually designated N) to give the *mean of the squared deviations* from the mean — usually just referred to as the *variance*. The reason the numbers are squared is to eliminate the problem of negative numbers which would arise since some of the numbers in the sample would be larger than the mean (hence subtracting them from the mean would give a negative result).

Exercise 4.3

What other problem would arise if we simply subtracted each number from the mean and added all the results? Try it to find out.

A problem with the variance is that having squared the numbers before adding them, we obtain quite a large figure which does not seem appropriate to the size of figures we're dealing with. For this reason (and others) the variance is often converted to a second measure of variability, the *standard deviation* by the simple expedient of taking the square root of the variance. The standard deviation provides an estimate of the variability which is in the same terms as the mean itself and which can be used to good effect in a number of other calculations.

In practice, calculating the standard deviation as described above can be tedious, particularly if dealing with several decimal places. The following formula gives identical results and is in most cases easier to use (even though it may look complicated!);

$$\frac{\sqrt{\sum x^2 - \frac{\left(\sum x\right)^2}{N}}}{N}$$

The symbol surrounding the equation is of course the familiar square root sign. The letters '*x*' and '*N*' refer to the numbers in the sample and the size of the sample respectively (thus you will have *N* of the *x*'s) and the $\sum$ character directs you to add together the numbers following the symbol, (the squares of *x* the first time it occurs, and the individual *x*'s the next time it occurs). Note that these two expressions $\sum x^2$ and $(\sum x)^2$ mean different things

— the first means "square each x and add the results" and the second means "add each x and square the result".

In the same way that the mean of a sample can be used to estimate the mean of a larger population, so can the standard deviation be used to estimate the variability of the larger population. When using the standard deviation for this purpose it has been found that a slight modification (called "Bessel's correction") leads to better estimates. The modification consists of replacing the final division by N with division by N-1. The revised formula therefore looks like this;

$$\frac{\sqrt{\sum x^2 - \frac{(\sum x)^2}{N}}}{N-1}$$

Thus we have a number of ways of estimating the variability of the data in which we are interested. With such an estimate of how much the data vary we are now in a position to estimate how likely we are to obtain certain values in our samples, and in particular how likely it is that samples we take would differ by a given amount purely by chance.

The Logic Of Significance Testing

We are now in a position to explore the logic underlying *significance testing*, a statistical approach which has come to dominate the way in which we make inferences from our data. The logic goes something like this:

i We can start out with two hypothesis options as described earlier; the *null hypothesis* (H_0), that there are no *real* differences between our variables, any apparent relationship being simply a result of random variation in our data, and an *alternative hypothesis* (H_1), that our variables *are* related to some extent.

ii Knowing something about the variability of our data enables us to say something about how likely certain apparent effects are likely to be even when only chance factors are operating. Thus if we toss a coin twice we may have two hypotheses; H_0 that the coin is a fair coin, and H_1 that it is in some way biased. If we obtain two heads from our two tosses, knowing how the results of coin tosses vary enables us to say that our result would occur with a probability of 0.25. Even if our null hypothesis were true — that is to say, repeating our experiment (two tosses) a large number of times, we would obtain a 'heads twice' result on roughly 25% of the occasions. Thus for this experiment, using a fair coin and deciding to conclude that it's biased if we obtain two heads would mean we would be wrong 25% of the time.

iii We can then say how often we are willing to be mistaken in rejecting our null hypothesis. Conventionally scientists have accepted certain standards in deciding to reject a null hypothesis or not. If the results we obtain are sufficiently rare that they would only occur by chance less than one in a hundred times, we reject the null hypothesis. Using such a strategy we will mistakenly reject such hypotheses only 1% of the time. In some contexts as we used in Chapter 3, a more lenient level of probability may be set. In this case a null hypothesis will be rejected if the results would occur by chance more than five in a hundred times. Using such a strategy we will of course reject the null hypothesis mistakenly more often (5% of the time rather than 1%). This is offset by the fact that we will be less likely to go along mistakenly *with* the null hypothesis when there really is in fact a relationship.

iv Note that if our data *do not* turn out to be particularly inconsistent with a chance interpretation, this does not mean that we've *proved* that chance factors are all that are operating. Often the data will be equally consistent with a chance hypothesis and an alternative hypothesis. Being unable to reject a null hypothesis means just that — that we can't rule out chance as an explanation. Nor, however, can we rule out other hypotheses — the question remains open.

v Because of the variety of the experimental questions we ask, most of which are more complicated than the coin-tossing example quoted above, specific statistical tests have been devised to enable us to interpret from various kinds of data how likely they would be to occur by chance. On this basis if the results do not seem particularly consistent with a chance interpretation, the null hypothesis can be rejected and an alternative explanation sought.

Student's T-Test; An Example Of A Statistical Test

We are now in a position to return to our original question of deciding whether or not the results we obtained earlier in the chapter can be seen as indicative of a *real* difference between the two groups or whether the differences we obtained could simply be a results of the chance variability in the populations from which we drew our samples.

One of the (relatively) simple ways of helping decide whether a difference in the means of two samples reflects a 'real' difference is by means of Student's t-test. The test was devised by W.S. Gosset, who modestly published his work under the non de plume 'Student' (hence the name of the test). For comparing two samples like the ones under consideration the formula is as follows;

$$t = \frac{\bar{x}_1 - \bar{x}_2}{\sqrt{\frac{\left(\sum x_1^2\right) - N_1\bar{x_1}^2 + \left(\sum x_2^2\right) - N_2\bar{x_2}^2}{N_1 + N_2 - 2}\left(\frac{1}{N_1} + \frac{1}{N_2}\right)}}$$

Although this looks complicated, if taken a little at a time it actually turns out to be quite simple. The figure being calculated, *t*, is termed a *statistic*. Its value is that for any pair of sample sizes we can calculate the probability of obtaining a t statistic higher (or lower) than a certain value. This, if we know what values are only likely to occur by chance less than once in a hundred times, we are able to say if the value we obtained is consistent with a chance interpretation.

We can illustrate the calculation and the use of t with the figures we started with in Table 4.1. Taking the individual items in the equation we have;

$\bar{x}_1,\ \bar{x}_2$	These are simply the mean values for groups 1 and 2 respectively; for our samples the values are 4.0 and 6.5.

$\left(\sum x_2^1\right), \left(\sum x_2^2\right)$ These values are taken by squaring each value and then totalling the results for groups 1 and 2 respectively. For our samples the results are 172 and 445.

$\bar{x}_1^2, \bar{x}_2^2$ These are simply the squares of the mean values for each group; for our samples the values are 16 and 42.25 respectively.

N_1, N_2 These are the sample sizes of groups 1 and 2 respectively; for our samples each is equal to 10.

Thus, substituting the above values in the equation above, we obtain;

$$t = \frac{4.0 - 6.5}{\frac{\sqrt{175 - 10(4^2) + 445 - 10(6.5^2)}}{10 + 10 - 2} \left(\frac{1}{10} + \frac{1}{10}\right)}$$

Simplifying this gives us;

$$t = \frac{-2.5}{\frac{\sqrt{172 - 160 + 445 - 442.5}}{18} \left(\frac{1}{5}\right)}$$

$$t = \frac{-2.5}{\sqrt{\frac{34.5}{90}}} = \frac{-2.5}{0.619} = -4.04$$

This figure, −4.04, is the *t-statistic* calculated for our data. It can be thought of as a single figure which summarises the essential information of the data relating to our original question — "is there a difference between the two groups?" For the t statistic (and for other statistics calculated to answer other questions) tables have been prepared which enable us to say whether the probability of obtaining such a figure from the samples we take is greater than or less than a particular level. As mentioned earlier we conventionally take probability levels of less than .05 or less than .01 as indicating that a chance interpretation of our results is implausible. That is to say, if the results we are obtaining would only occur by chance once in a hundred times, or five times in a hundred, we are inclined to *reject* our null hypothesis (that the effect is purely a chance effect) and instead conclude that there really is some difference in the two populations from which our samples have been drawn.

Using The T Statistic And Appropriate Tables

In order to use the result of our calculations to draw a conclusion, it is necessary to consult tables of the t statistic. These can be found in standard statistical textbooks but the following table shows the relevant information.

Table 4.3: 'Students' *t*-distribution

Degrees of Freedom	Value of *P*		
	0.05	0.01	0.001
10	2.23	3.17	4.59
18	2.10	2.88	3.92
20	1.72	2.84	3.85

In cases like the one under consideration we need to know the number of *degrees of freedom* in the two samples and the calculated *t*-statistic. The number of degrees of freedom, for this statistic, is obtained by subtracting 1 from each of the sample sizes. That is to say, in the present example we have 18 (9+9) degrees of freedom. Consulting a table of the t-statistic reveals that any *absolute* value of t (one ignoring whether it is positive or negative) greater than 2.88 from samples having 18 degrees of freedom is likely to occur by chance less than once in a hundred times. Such a result is described as being *significant* with a probability of less than .01, usually referred to as "significant at the .01 level". Since our results would be unlikely to occur by chance, we conclude that the null hypothesis is unacceptable as an explanation of our findings and reject it. A result such as this is usually written;

$$t = -4.04, \quad 18df, p < .01$$

meaning that the value of the statistic is 4.04, there are 18 degrees of freedom, and that such a result would occur by change in less than a hundred times. If the result had *not* been significant, a probability value would not usually be quoted, but the figure would simply be described as 'not significant' (often abbreviated to NS).

Degrees of Freedom

The concept of degrees of freedom is a complex one in statistics, and relates to the amount of information in each item of data. In principle you can think of the degrees of freedom as the number of data items which could vary and still leave the sole sample with certain relevant characteristics. In our present case the mean is the feature of the samples which cannot vary for the question we are asking. Thus, for a sample of ten people, the first nine can take any value they wish, but the tenth would then be determined if we were to end up with the same mean value. Putting this another way, nine of the sample can vary as much as they like; this is described by saying that the sample has *nine* degrees of freedom.

For most simple calculations the degrees of freedom can be specified in some simple way — in this case the degrees of freedom for each sample is one less than the sample size, i.e. is equal to N-1.

One- And Two-Tailed Tests And The Interpretation Of Statistical Tables

Statistical tables will typically give probability values associated with the value of the relevant statistic in two forms; those for *one-tailed* tests and those for *two-tailed* tests. For most purposes the values given for two-tailed tests will be those that are required. A one-tailed test is only used when there is knowledge beforehand that the relationship being sought could only take one form. Thus, if we could argue that it was *impossible* that the group from which our first sample was drawn could have a higher mean than the group from which our second sample was drawn. We do not consider two possible outcomes — whether our first group is significantly greater than the second and whether it is significantly less. We need consider only whether it is significantly less. Even if our *samples* had been such that the first had appeared to be significantly higher than the second, we still wouldn't reject the null hypothesis because we started out *knowing* that the first could not really be greater than the second. Under these circumstances only one extreme (or 'tail') of the whole range of possible values is of interest. When this is the case, the cutoff value for regarding a result in the 'right' direction will be less stringent than if either extreme would be possible. You can think of this as being rather like a deal. In return for agreeing not to reject the null hypothesis for extreme values in one direction, you are given permission to reject it for rather more lenient values in the other.

You should note that it can be very difficult to make a case for using a one-tailed rather then a two-tailed test. It is very hard to claim that it would be nonsense for a result to turn out in one direction but not in the other, and some statisticians would argue that one-tailed tests should *never* be used. For example, it might be tempting to think that it wouldn't make sense for a group given a medicine for some illness to do better than one not given the medicine — but it is not *impossible* (the harmful effects of the medicine might outweigh the benefits).

In general you will probably find it most useful to interpret your results in the context of two-tailed tests. Whilst it can be frustrating, on occasions, to obtain results which are significant on a one-tailed test but not on a two-tailed, you should not use a one-tailed test unless you are *absolutely* certain that it is justified.

Some Caveats Regarding The T-Test

Not surprisingly a relatively complex procedure like the t-test leaves open a number of possibilities for making mistakes. The test makes a number of assumptions. Some of these can be violated without too much trouble, but others are crucial. The assumptions include;

i. The two samples must be independent. In our example, the sampling of the first group had no effect on the sampling of the second. The most important situation in which this is not the case is when each member of the first group stands in some relationship to a particular member of the second. Thus, if each person in group two were the mother of a particular individual in group one, the two groups would not be independent. The same problem arises if we have groups in which the members of one are the spouses of the others, when each member of a second group is 'matched' to a member of the first in one or more respects (e.g. age) or when the second group consists of a second measure taken on the same individuals present in the first group. In these cases a variant of the t-test called the *related t-test* or *paired t-test* should be used. For this reason the test we have described is sometimes referred to as the *unrelated* or *unpaired* t-test. This assumption is one of the ones which should *never* be violated.

ii. The observations within each sample must be independent. Thus, if the sample were obtained by asking each subject to nominate the next subject there is the risk that this second person might be more like the first than an individual chosen at random. Clearly this would have implications for the overall mean calculated for that sample and for the estimate of variability. For the most part this assumption should be thought of as one which it is unsafe to violate.

iii. The observations should be drawn from populations which themselves have similar variances. In practice the two variances can differ by a fairly reasonable amount before the results are substantially affected. Conscientious researchers (and many computerised statistical programs) can test the significance of differences between the two variances in order to check this assumption.

iv. The observations should be drawn from populations which are *normally* distributed. The 'normal' (or Gaussian) distribution is a pattern of distribution of scores which looks something like the cross section of a bell, with a peak in the middle falling off symmetrically to each side. In practice as long as the populations from which the samples are drawn are reasonably symmetrical (the mean, mode and median being roughly similar) then deviations from strict normality are unlikely to have a very marked effect on the results obtained.

The Mann-Whitney U Test

Amongst the assumptions underlying the Student's t-test was that the observations should come from distributions which are at least *approximately* normal. Although slight deviations from this assumption seem to make little or no difference to the results of the test, the distributions may sometimes be so extreme as to make the assumption unreasonable. Statisticians have devised a range of tests known as *nonparametric* or *distribution-free* tests to cope with such situations. The nearest nonparametric equivalent to Student's t-test is the Mann-Whitney U test. This tests a slightly different null hypothesis to the t-test; where the t-test's null hypothesis is that the two samples have the same *mean*, the Mann-Whitney U test is that the samples have the same *median*.

The 'Power' of a Test

At first glance it might seem sensible to use nonparametric tests all the time, since they make fewer assumptions than their parametric equivalents. Perhaps unsurprisingly, however, there are disadvantages as well as advantages to using nonparametric tests. In general nonparametric tests are less *powerful* than parametric ones. Here less powerful means that for any given probability of a Type I error a nonparametric test will have a higher probability than a parametric one of a Type II error.

Summary

1. Experimental plans are best stated in the form of null or alternative hypotheses.

2. Type I and Type II errors consider ways in which conclusions can be drawn.

3. The variability of the data will indicate the likelihood of the results occurring by chance.

4. The t-test is one method of examining whether or not there is a real difference between tests. It is examined in detail including the degrees of freedom and the levels of significance.

5. Two-tailed tests are the most commonly used with one-tailed tests when there is advance knowledge that the relationship being sought could only take one form.

6. The t-test involves a number of assumptions including that the observations should be drawn from populations which are normally distributed.

7. The Mann-Whitney U test is the nearest nonparametric equivalent to the t-test.

CHAPTER 5

EXPERIMENTS WITH ONE OR A FEW SUBJECTS

Key words : *ABA design; ABAB design; placebo; changing interior design; reversal designs; multiple baseline designs; replication; serial dependency; autocorrelation; time series analysis.*

Introduction

So far we have concentrated on large groups but there is often a case in the health sciences to study not groups of subjects but individuals.

The experimental study of single cases has a long history in the biological and psychological sciences. Note that here we are not talking about the 'case history' (which itself has a valuable role in science) but rather about the intensive experimental study of single individuals. The argument is a simple one. Rather than obtaining large groups of individuals in the hope that the differences between them will average out revealing differences in treatment or training, why not just study the individual, so that such differences do not arise in the first place?

Of course over the years it has become clear that the picture is far from simple, and indeed the original notion of 'single subject research' has now been subsumed under a broader heading of *'small-N research'* i.e. research involving only small samples. The essential characteristic of such research is that the use of derived statistics is kept to a minimum, with concentration on the results of each individual subject in a study. In doing so aspects of a phenomenon which would remain undetected using conventional designs may become apparent.

Perhaps the most widespread application of small-N research designs has been in behavioural psychology. Many early experiments in behavioural psychology involved the study of simple behaviours repeated over long periods of time, with various experimental interventions introduced in order to examine their effects on the behaviour in question (e.g. Skinner 1938; Ferster and Skinner 1957). One of the first textbooks specifically concerned with the logic and methods of small-N research was specifically concerned with the applications of the approach to behavioural experiments (Sidman 1960). Subsequent application of the methods and principles of behavioural psychology to clinical problems led to the development and refinement of these methods for the study of clinical problems.

Methods Of Small-N Research

The ABA design

The simplest method used in small-N research is the so-called 'ABA' design. Whilst simple, it illustrates a number of the important principles of such research. The term 'ABA' refers to the phases of the experiment being conducted. During the initial 'A' phase, data are collected in the absence of any experimental manipulation. Thus, in an experiment to investigate the effect of various experimental procedures on pulse rate, the 'A' phase might involve taking the pulse of the subject before the experiment starts. In such a case it is advantageous to repeat such a measure on several occasions — perhaps at intervals of every two minutes. In this way the natural variation in pulse rate over time for that individual can be determined. Such data are referred to as 'baseline' data, and in most cases moving onto the second ('B') phase of the experiment will not take place until a stable baseline has been achieved. Obtaining a stable baseline means that it is considerably easier to interpret any subsequent changes; if pulse rate varies by only one or two beats per minute during the baseline phase, an increase of twenty beats per minute cannot be explained in terms of the simple moment to moment variation.

Having obtained a reasonably stable baseline the experimental manipulation can be introduced. For example, the subject may be required to perform five minutes of sustained exercise; the pulse can again be read at intervals throughout the exercise and such readings continued when the exercise finishes. If you conduct such an experiment you will find that after a short time the baseline readings of the individual's pulse become reasonably stable; during exercise they rise and then following exercise (the return to the baseline conditions) the readings return to around their original level. Such a study provides a simple demonstration of the way in which heart rate is (in part) a function of level of activity.

Whilst simple in concept and execution, such a methodology is not without its limitations. Firstly it should be noted that there is some risk of confounding factors; if for example you try doing this experiment on yourself, it could be argued that the rise in your pulse is a result not of actually doing the exercise but of *deciding* to do the exercise. On the other hand, if someone else has decided when to move from the baseline phase to the experimental phase such an explanation would not hold. A second problem is that there is likely to be some time lag between the changes of experimental phase and the effect being apparent in the data. For example, it may take a little time for pulse rate to rise during exercise, and similarly it may take time for the pulse to return to normal when returning to the baseline conditions. A third, and perhaps more severe problem, is that there remains the possibility that the change in experimental conditions and the change in pulse rate is coincidental, and that it was really some other change happening at the same time as the change in activity which was really responsible. Finally there is the problem that if the purpose of the experiment was to *produce* some change in performance (for example if one were investigating different ways of improving athletic ability) the design leaves the subject exactly where she or he started.

The latter problems have led to the consideration by researchers within a small-N paradigm of issues of repeated measurement. The result has been a number of extensions of the basic ABA design, intended to provide a greater degree of confidence in the interpretation of results.

The ABAB design

The ABAB design, as its name suggests, extend the ABA design by repeating not only the baseline conditions but also the experimental phase. By introducing an experimental phase on two occasions, the possibility of obtaining a change by coincidental change in other factors is directly reduced. Assuming that the decision on when to introduce the second experimental phases is taken appropriately the probability of their coinciding with some other change is halved. Moreover, since the design ends in the intervention phase, this means that any attempt to investigate therapeutic or educational change in this way can leave such changes in operation at the end of the study.

It is easy to see how our previous example of an ABA design showing the link between heart rate and exercise could be extended to an ABAB design — all that would be necessary would be a second exercise phase to demonstrate again that it was indeed the change in activity that was associated with the change in pulse. Perhaps a closer parallel to the clinical applications would be one in which the effects of a particular technique were to be demonstrated in sports performance. For example in the discus throw, pressing down on the discus with the thumb of the throwing hand can help in imparting a spin to the discus and thereby improve performance. For a novice discus thrower it would be possible to measure the distance thrown with and without such a technique as the B and A phases respectively of an ABAB design. On this basis it would be possible to determine whether or not this particular technique was in fact helping the competitor in question.

In practice of course the use of such experimental techniques requires rather more skill and consideration than might initially be apparent. In most practical situations there may be a number of problems to be surmounted. Especially important in many cases is the difficulty of obtaining a stable baseline. For example, in the evaluation of particular techniques in discus throwing described above, the likelihood is that during the baseline phase the distances thrown by the experimental subject will be quite variable. Some factors, like the increasing experience as the baseline phase proceeds, will tend to increase the distance thrown. Others (e.g. tiredness) will tend to decrease it. Whilst some of these problems can be circumvented directly, (e.g. by leaving sufficiently long rest periods for the athlete to recover) others may be more problematic. Figure 5.1 shows what a desirable baseline can look like and illustrates some of the problems that may be encountered in obtaining a stable baseline;

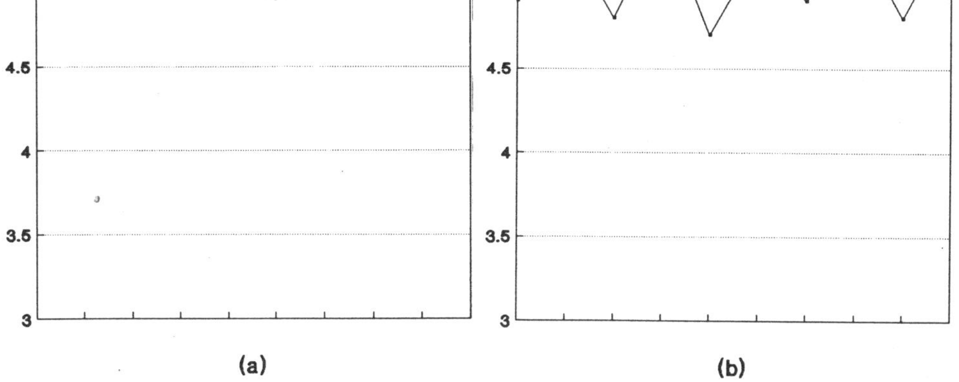

Figure 5.1 Types of baselines

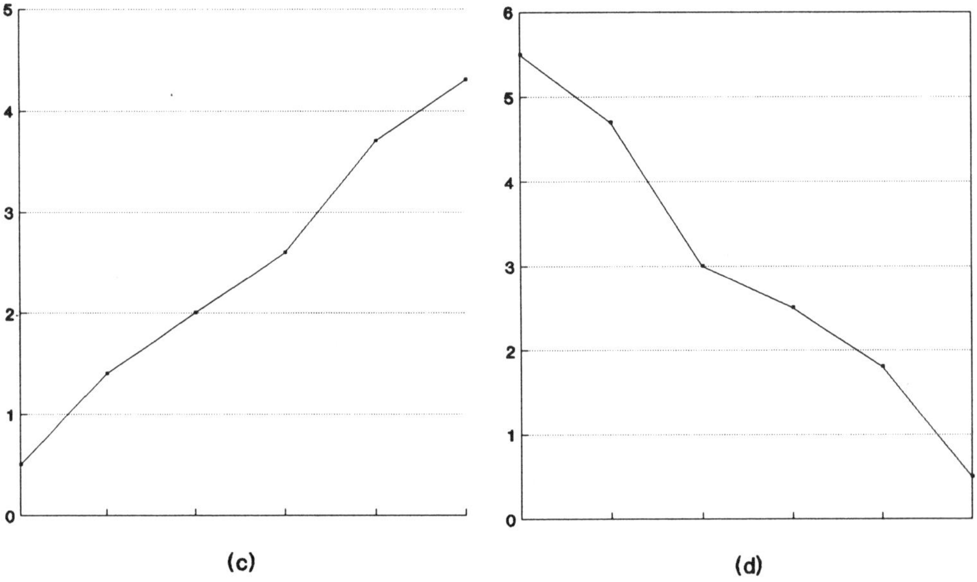

Figure 5.1 (continued) : Types of baselines

Figure 5.1(a) shows the kind of baseline that makes an ABAB experiment easy; the variation is only slight and there is no evidence of any systematic trend in the variation that is apparent. Figure 5.1(b) on the other hand is considerably less stable. Here the results of successive trials are extremely variable, and it could be difficult to detect any change in the data when the experimental phase begins. Under these circumstances the experimenter has at least two immediate courses of action open. The first is simply to continue the baseline measurements in the hope that they eventually settle down. Alternatively, the experimenter can reason that the variability in the data reflect some factor that is varying from trial to trial and which is producing massive swings in the results of each trial. The discus thrower may sometimes be looking down at the moment of the throw and sometimes be looking up, or there may be some external factor like dramatic changes in the prevailing wind. By identifying factors which are producing the variation the experimenter can take steps to control them or eliminate their effects — for example by instructing the subject to look up on every occasion, or by measuring the wind velocity and direction and only permitting trials when these are within certain limits.

To a certain degree these problems and solutions also apply with the baselines shown in figures 5.1(c) and 5.1(d) which show clear trends up and down. Such trends might not of course be a major problem; if the experimenter is confident, for example, that the experimental procedure will produce a dramatic improvement in performance, this may contrast so markedly with the previous downward trend that the effect is obvious. On the other hand, if the trend had already been up, critics might wish to argue that any further improvement in performance is simply a continuation of the existing trend rather than an effect of the intervention. Conversely, if the initial trend had been down, it might be difficult to demonstrate any improvement if such improvement is being cancelled out by the prevailing downward trend.

It is generally a good idea to obtain the most stable baseline possible before implementing any experimental change; often the experimenter will have some idea of the size of effect likely to result from the intervention (or, in many practical settings, the minimum effect that would be worthwhile) and can therefore determine whether the baseline is sufficiently stable relative to the size of effect expected to permit an effect to be demonstrated.

Having obtained a sufficiently stable baseline, there remain a number of important considerations. For example, having taken a certain number of trials to obtain a stable baseline (A), how long should the experimental phase (B) last? This question has been discussed by a number of authors, most notably Hersen and Barlow (1976). At first glance it might be tempting to argue that the experimental phase should last as long as is necessary to obtain a stable baseline. In general, however, such 'real time' decision making on phase length is to be discouraged. Apart from anything else, there is the real danger that an experimenter shows unconscious bias in deciding that a phase should end when the desired results have been obtained. There is some evidence (e.g. Rosenthal 1964) that unless precautions are taken to prevent such bias, it can result in seriously misleading results. Deciding before the data are gathered how long the experimental phase will last is one way of defending against such a problem.

In discussing this issue, Hersen and Barlow (1976) argue that for most purposes it is advisable that baseline and experimental phases should include similar or equal numbers of data points. Thus, if fifteen pulse measurements were taken in the baseline phase in the experiment described above, then fifteen measurements should be taken in the experimental phase, the second baseline and the second experimental phase, making a total of sixty measurements in all. Of course, having decided in advance that the two experimental phases (B) and the second baseline (A) are all to be the same length as the first baseline (A) the possibility arises that these last three phases may not show sufficient stability in the data. This may be a particular problem where any form of 'carryover' effect is apparent from phase to phase. For example if changing the conditions of the experiment from baseline to experiment confuses the subject causing temporary disruption of behaviour, or if the effects of the preceding phase persist into the succeeding one (for example if an increase in heart rate takes some time to recover). To a certain extent these problems can be overcome if the extent and duration of such carryover can be estimated in advance. It is unlikely that much of the increase in pulse over ten minutes exercise will still be apparent after an hour, so scheduling the second baseline phase for an hour after the completion of the experimental phase should avoid most carryover effects. It can of course be argued that carryover is an important part of a transition, that it should itself be part of the study. In this case the experimenter might wish to run all phases consecutively in order that the pattern of change from one level of activity to another might be studied.

A more detailed discussion of the problems of determining phase length can be found in Hersen and Barlow (1976) who draw attention to other factors which may need to be taken into account (e.g. cyclical factors; an ABAB design which allocated a week to each phase might run into problems with female subjects whose menstrual cycle could affect the results. Other cyclical factors might be external, such as seasonal effects in long-term studies or even differences between weekends and weekdays). Many other problems of ABAB designs can be addressed using extensions or variants of such procedures. For the basic ABAB design, however, the essential stages can be summarised as follows:

i. Suitable independent and dependent variables should be selected (e.g. activity level and pulse rate).

ii. Scheduling of the phases should be planned as far as possible to take account of the need to obtain stable baselines. Allow for carryover and transition from one phase to the next and avoid cyclical effects. In some cases it may be necessary to gather preliminary data regarding the amount of stability that can be expected during baseline and taking suitable action (e.g. controlling confounding factors) if necessary.

iii. Data should be gathered throughout the phases of the experiment, ensuring as far as possible that there is no systematic difference between phases except that which defines them; thus in the experiment above, the only difference between the A and B phases should be the level of activity. It would be a mistake for example to have one researcher taking the pulse measurements during the baseline phases and a different experimenter doing so during the experimental phases.

iv. Usually the data from such experiments will be presented in simple graphical form showing the difference in level of the dependent variable in the four phases. Under some circumstances a degree of statistical analysis may be considered; careful consideration is needed here of the appropriateness of such statistics and some of the issues involved are discussed later in this chapter.

Simple extensions of the ABAB design

Under some circumstances we may wish to include more than the basic four phases of the ABAB design into our studies. Perhaps the most obvious of these is when we wish to investigate more than one kind of experimental procedure. For example, in the study of effects of exercise on pulse rate we might wish to investigate and compare the effects of both isokinetic and isotonic exercise, or of the effects of different intensities of exercise. Such a problem can be addressed in a number of ways. If we call the first experimental procedure (e.g. isokinetic exercise) B_1 and the second B_2 we could extend the design to forms such as $AB_1AB_2AB_1AB_2A$, or to $AB_1AB_1AB_2AB_2$ (the latter is of course equivalent to running two separate ABAB experiments one after the other, the first using the experimental condition number one and the second experimental condition number two) or to various other combinations. Often decisions regarding the various permutations of this kind will depend on a range of factors including logistical ones like how much time is available and theoretical ones like the extent to which the effects of one phase can be expected to interfere with another.

A design which is in many ways formally equivalent to the kind of extension described in the preceding paragraph has been described by Hersen and Barlow (1976) as an ABCB design. In this the second baseline phase is not a return to the conditions prevailing before the experiment began, but is instead a maintenance of the experimental conditions but without a specific factor considered to be crucial. Of particular relevance in clinical research, this substitutes for the second baseline a phase designed to take account of non-specific factors in the intervention such as the placebo effect or the 'Hawthorne effect'.

Placebo and Hawthorn Effects

One of the common problems encountered by researchers is that the very act of conducting the research can have an effect on the subject under study. This problem of *reflexivity* has been described in a number of contexts. At the simple level, we are confronted with the fact that people may behave differently simply because they are being observed; the Hawthorne effect was named after a study attempting to assess the effects of different level of illumination on worker productivity, when it was found that the very act of conducting the research produced improvements, presumably by making the subjects feel in some way special. The problem has been particularly important in the study of effects of drugs, where it has been found that even when people are given a substance with no medicinal properties whatever (a *placebo*) a percentage of subjects will show some degree of improvement (and may even do so if they are *told* that the 'drug' has no properties!). Clearly any attempt to assess the effects of a drug has to allow for such a placebo effect, and a drug needs to show that it produces a better effect than a placebo for it to be considered useful.

In an ABCB design, the C phase typically consists of exactly the same procedure as the B phase with the removal of the experimental element felt to be essential. This can be illustrated in the context of the hypothetical study of the effects of exercise on behaviour. In a simple ABAB design, the individual might first have a series of pulse measurements taken, then be taken to a gymnasium to exercise on a cycle ergometer during the experimental phase, taken back to a rest room during the second baseline phase and then required to repeat the activity during the second experimental phase. In an ABCB design the second baseline might not require the subject to return to a rest room but might instead involve remaining on the cycle ergometer but without any work being done. In such an example, the difference between the two designs begins to look very much like one of variation in degree of experimental control. The ABCB design is perhaps of most importance in clinical research, where a particular drug or treatment is being tested. Here baseline data may be gathered before any drug at all is used, but the C phase may not involve a return to baseline conditions but rather the replacement of the active drug with a placebo. In a health context a similar strategy might for example be used to assess the value of a treatment like hypnosis; measures of performance could be taken before treatment began, and then a C phase could be implemented in which the psychologist continued to see the patient but provided no hypnosis. In this way it would be possible to evaluate the benefits of hypnosis whilst making due allowance for any benefits which simply resulted from receiving the interested attentions of a relevant professional.

The kinds of designs we have so far been discussing come under the general heading of *reversal* designs. That is to say, they involve, at some point, reversing the procedures of the previous phase in order to obtain a return to the baseline (or, as in the ABCB and similar designs, a modified baseline). This issue of reversal highlights one of the most obvious limitations of this kind of study — the fact that it is not always *possible* to reverse some experimental condition. This is perhaps most obvious in instances where the experimental phase involves some imparting of information. If we want to look at the effect of knowledge on performance of some task, it is difficult to see how we can take back any information we have given to the subject in order to implement a second baseline. In some circumstances (e.g. certain therapeutic interventions) it may be possible but undesirable to revert to a baseline condition. For problems of this kind it is necessary to go beyond the reversal design. One such extension is that known as the *changing criterion* design. As with many of the designs described here this was originally devised in the context of applied behavioural psychology. It does however have applications beyond such a setting. In the changing criterion design baseline data are set and an intervention applied as in a simple AB design. However, once stable responding has been obtained in the B phase this is then used as the baseline for a further intervention. In the original context of the changing criterion design some change in behaviour would be specified as necessary in order to achieve a particular outcome (e.g. some form of reward). Once the change in behaviour had been achieved and stabilized the criterion for achieving the reward would be made slightly more stringent. This procedure could then be extended until a substantial change in behaviour had been produced. A similar procedure might be of interest in some sporting contexts. For example, a judo player taught a new technique might be required to compete only against opponents of limited skill. Once these could be regularly defeated, opponents of a higher level of ability could be fought, the level of competence of the opposition being increased each time the ability to defeat current opponents stabilised. Such a technique is of course widely used in practical coaching but can also form the basis of an experimental procedure for demonstrating the effectiveness of the particular technique.

In practice the use of the changing criterion design involves a number of problems, and its applicability will often be limited. The fact that it is not always possible to reverse a treatment phase thus remains a problem for ABA designs and their various extensions. As a result a further class of procedures has been developed to deal with such problems — the multiple baseline design.

Multiple baseline designs

Multiple baseline approaches to small-N research were first developed in the context of applied behavioural psychology. A typical problem might concern attempts to modify self-injurious behaviour of psychiatric patients. Clearly there are problems here in suggesting any form of reversal, since if at the end of the first experimental phase there has been a reduction in such behaviour there would be serious ethical problems in suggesting a return to baseline conditions. The problem is similar when the behaviour in question is one which whilst not harmful to the patient may be harmful to others.

The basic principle of the multiple baseline design is that, as the name suggest, baselines are taken on several independent measures — almost always in this context several different behaviours. The proposed intervention is then applied to just one of the behaviours whilst baseline data continue to be collected on the others. If the provision of the intervention has a demonstrable effect on the first behaviour, it is then applied to the second, whilst baseline data continue to be gathered on the remaining behaviours. Gradually the process is repeated until a change in all of the behaviours has been demonstrated by the successive implementation of the intervention.

The practical implementation of the multiple-baseline procedure is perhaps best illustrated in the context of the kinds of problem with which it was first demonstrated. For example, in a study by Cooke and Apolloni (1976) children with a learning disability were taught four discrete behaviours — smiling, sharing, positive physical contact and verbal complimenting. A combination of procedures was used to teach these behaviours, including demonstrating the behaviour and providing instructions and praise. Thus for one subject (Subject number 2) baseline data were collected on all four behaviours; after nine sessions of collecting baseline data attempts were made to increase sharing behaviour whilst continuing to collect baseline data on the other three behaviours. Over the next five sessions sharing was shown to increase whilst the remaining three behaviours continued at much the same level as before. In later phases of the experiment smiling, positive physical contact and verbal complimenting were successively taught. For each the baseline level of performance remained low until the training programme for that particular behaviour began. It was thus possible to show for four different behaviours that the change in frequency of the behaviour was directly associated with the introduction of the training programme. If only one behaviour had been selected, it would have been possible to argue that the changes in the behaviour were possibly due to some other, unknown, event coincidental with the start of the programme. It is unlikely however that for each of the behaviours any such change would be both specific in its effects to the particular behaviour under study. Remember that the other behaviours remained unaltered whilst their baseline data were being collected. The hypothesised coincidental event would occur every time just as the training programme were started. It was thus possible to demonstrate clearly that the changes in behaviour were indeed a function of the training programme without having to resort to any reversal of behaviour. This could have been difficult, as mentioned earlier, as the instructions could not reasonably have been 'withdrawn'.

Barlow and Hersen (1984) distinguish three types of multiple baseline design. The multiple baseline across behaviours (as described above) where several behaviours are sequentially subject to the experimental manipulation, usually within a single subject; multiple baseline across subjects, where (usually) a single type of behaviour is monitored across several subjects, the experimental intervention being introduced at different times for the various subjects; and multiple baselines across settings, where an experimental manipulation is applied (usually to a single behaviour with a single subject) sequentially in a range of various settings. This latter approach is perhaps most relevant in the clinical setting where attempts are made to change behaviour which is being maintained by some environmental contingency. For example, it may be felt that a problem behaviour is occurring because of the attention it generates from others. In an across-settings multiple baseline design the behaviour may be monitored in a variety of settings (at home, at school etc.) and changes made in the amount of contingent attention provided in these settings. If the behaviour becomes less frequent in each setting only as the amount of attention provided changes in each setting, this provides strong evidence that the behaviour is indeed a function of the attention.

The basic procedure of the multiple baseline design can therefore be summarised as follows;

i. Determine which of the three broad types of multiple baseline design is to be used (in practice a design may involve permutations of all three — for example monitoring several behaviours of several subjects in various settings).

ii. Gather baseline data on all of the behaviours/subject/settings until a stable baseline is obtained.

iii. Introduce the experimental manipulation to one of the behaviours/subjects/settings whilst continuing to gather baseline data on the rest.

iv. After a period of time (probably best determined in advance, possibly a period equal to the initial baseline) introduce the experimental manipulation to the second of the behaviours/subjects/settings. Again continuing to gather baseline data on the remainder and further experimental data on the first behaviour/subject/setting.

v. Continue the procedure until the last of the behaviours/subjects/settings has completed its experimental phase.

Clearly for a multiple baseline design to be effective it is important that the behaviours involved are independent. Consider for example what would happen if we attempted to use a within-subjects multiple baseline design to investigate the effects of weight training on athletic throwing events. We might take baselines on an athlete's ability in shot, discus and javelin and then introduce a weight training programme for the shot whilst continuing to monitor performance in the other two events. However, the three events are not completely independent, and weight training designed to be of benefit to one of the three will almost certainly have effects on the other two events as well. Thus, although the weight training might indeed produce improvements in the shot, it is likely that the weight programme for the shot would also produce benefits in the discus and javelin (even if these were not as great as for the shot). An attempt to conduct a within-subjects multiple baseline (or indeed a between settings multiple baseline) would therefore fail since *all* the baselines would improve once the weight training started. It would therefore be impossible to claim that the improvement was indeed a result of the weight training and not of some unknown coincidental change taking place at the same time. Any attempt to use a multiple baseline design to investigate this problem would therefore require the use of more than one subject and hence a between-subjects multiple baseline design. That is to say, baselines would be taken from several subjects performance in the throwing events and then a weight training programme would be introduced for the first whilst continuing to take baseline data on the remaining subjects. After a time the weight training would be introduced for the second, then the third and so on until the training had been introduced to all subjects.

Replication

Eagle-eyed readers will by now have noticed that the between subjects multiple baseline design, as described above, is little different to conducting a series of AB designs with a number of subjects one after another. Perhaps the only important difference is that in the multiple baseline design the baseline data begins to be gathered from each subject at the same time, even though the times of the interventions differ. This brings us to a central issue in the consideration of small-N designs, that of *replication*. In discussing large-group designs we have emphasised the benefits of taking large random samples in order that any results obtained may be generalized to the population of which the sample is felt to be representative. From this point of view the notion of conducting research on small sample sizes obviously raises immediate problems of generalizability. Of course in some situations this may not be a problem - the investigator may not wish to generalize beyond the particular individual being studied. This might be the case for example in a clinical situation where a therapist was attempting to study the problems of an individual patient, or in a coaching situation where a coach was attempting to improve the performance of a single athlete.

By and large, however, most researchers will probably want to feel that the findings of their studies will be generalizable to other individuals. For this reason most researchers will wish to *replicate* their findings with additional subjects. Such replication may take a number of forms. *Direct replication*, as its name implies, simply involves repeating the experiment with another subject. If the same results are obtained, another direct replication may be performed, and another, until the researcher is convinced that the finding really is generalizable across individuals.

Sidman (1960), author of what is probably the classic work on small-N research notes at least two other forms of replications. In *systematic replication*, the study is repeated but certain variables are deliberately altered from one replication to another. This might involve manipulation of subject variables, experimental variables, or both. Thus if a researcher had demonstrated a particular phenomenon or relationship with a male subject, the next demonstration might be conducted with a female subject. If the first had been with a young subject, the second might be with an older subject, and so on. If the effect persists in the face of such changes (a different subject of different age, sex etc) the experimenter learns something about the relationship between the effect and these variables - not least that the variables are not necessarily specific to one age group, or one sex. Similarly the experimenter may wish to change experimental variables. Having demonstrated the benefits of isotonic weight training on throwing performance with one subject, an attempt might be made to demonstrate a similar effect with isokinetic training with the next subject. Again, if the effect persists the experimenter has been able to demonstrate that the effect is not specific to one form of training. Thus with only two subjects the experimenter has been able to gain valuable information not only about the phenomenon but about the variables of which it may or may not be a function.

Sidman's second form of replication is that of *affirming the consequent*. Whilst conceding that this has "no foundation in logic" Sidman nevertheless argues that such replication is "the lifeblood of science". The principle of affirming the consequent can be thought of as systematic replication with practically *all* variables changed. A scientist affirming the consequent might argue in the example of the weight training/throwing experiment as follows; "The theory suggests that providing a specific training for that event will produce an improvement. My study has shown that power training with weights improves throwing events. This implication of the theory for endurance events is that specific cardiovascular training would be of benefit. I will therefore replicate my first confirmation of the theory (with the thrower) by conducting a second study with an endurance athlete, using a totally different form of training appropriate to this different event. If I once again see an improvement, this gives further support to the theory."

Of course, the discussion so far has optimistically assumed that the results of the original study will indeed be repeated in the replication. What however happens when the results fail to be replicated? Here too, thesmall-N researcher argues, the use of such designs has advantages over larger group studies. In the large group study, when a phenomenon fails to be consistently demonstrable across individuals, the best that the researcher can simply do is to quote an average (which we have seen at the beginning of the chapter may be totally unrepresentative of *any* individual) or to note the percentage of individuals in whom the phenomenon can be demonstrated. The small-N researcher, however with only a limited number of subjects, can quickly be on the trail of the relevant variables. If a replication fails, the experimenter can immediately note what differences there are between the original study and the replication. Were the experimental conditions similar or different? Did the type of training change? Was the subject the same sex, the same age, the same level of experience etc? Having studied intensively each of the subjects, the experimenter is immediately able to compile a 'shortlist' of possible causes for the failure to replicate. These can then be investigated directly in further studies. If for example the subject in the replication was a different sex to the original subject, a third subject the same sex as the original can be obtained; do the original results reappear? If so, what is it about being a different sex that accounts for the difference? Is it to do with physical strength? Is so, can a person of the same sex as the first subject but similar strength to the second be found? Whilst the large-group researcher is tediously sampling and averaging fifty or a hundred individuals, the small-N researcher is already well into the detective work of tracking down the relevant variables.

The argument can be continued beyond one of efficiency. Not only is the small-N researcher quickly able to start pursuing the variables which are causing the differences in the results, it can be argued that this is indeed the responsibility of the researcher. When an experimenter removes the effect of unwanted variability in a large group by averaging, it is argued, the very subject matter of the research is being lost. If something is causing such variability, then that source of variability *must* be tracked down and identified if the phenomenon is to be understood. In this sense the small-N researcher goes further than the experimenter with the large group, by not being content simply to *measure* variability but by tracking it's sources to understand and possibly control it.

From this viewpoint it becomes apparent that the approach to generality adopted by the small-N researcher is notably different from that of the researcher using large groups. For the latter, generalizability is an issue of representativeness of sampling. For the former, generalizability is an issue of having sufficient understand of the phenomenon in question to predict how it will be affected by a change in conditions. Putting it crudely, the large group researcher might simply take a representative sample of throwers from a population of athletes and assess the mean improvement produced by weight training. Confronted with a new athlete the researcher would then use this mean improvement as a 'best estimate' of how much improvement might be produced by the training. The small-N researcher however would argue that generalizing to this new subject requires understanding of the *process* by which weight training produces its benefits, and might determine (for example) that such a weight training programme would produce notable benefits in middle-ability athletes whose technique was reasonable but who lacked power, but would produce little benefit in beginners (who would be limited by technique irrespective of power) or top class athletes (who might already be training so hard that the influence of the additional weight training programme would be minimal). Thus, generalizability for the experimenter using large groups is an issue of *measuring* variability, using such measures to indicate limits to how much a phenomenon may change with new subjects, conditions, etc. For the experimenter using small-N designs generalizability is a matter of understanding the problem sufficiently to say how such changes will affect the phenomenon of interest.

Statistical Procedures And Small-N Designs

It will be recalled that in discussing large group statistical procedures (Chapter 4) the use of various statistical tests was outlined. Such tests form a basis for determining whether relationships apparent in data, differences between groups and so on could have arisen by chance or can be thought to reflect 'real' effects shown by the study. It is not difficult to see how similar questions might arise in small-N research. If, for example, we see differences between the A and B phases of our experiment, how can we tell if the difference is big enough to be sure it reflects a real effort and not just chance variation.

One answer might be to use the same kinds of tests we use with large group designs — t-test, analysis of variance and so on. It would be possible to regard the data in the A phase and the data in the B phase as two different groups, take the means of each group, and perform a t-test to determine whether the difference between them was significant. Unfortunately this turns out to be somewhat problematic. One of the assumptions underlying the kinds of tests we described in Chapter 4 is that each observation (and hence each data point) is associated with a certain amount of error (and hence variability). It is essential for the conduct of the statistical tests that such error be random, that is to say the error associated with one observation must not be associated with the error of the next. A moment's reflection will reveal why this is important. If we obtain two data points which are completely independent, each give us valuable information. If however the two data points were closely dependent (i.e. the error on the second could be predicted from the first) then we would be in a position, knowing the first data point, to make a very good guess at what the second would be; actually knowing what the second data point is would not therefore tell us very much. It's rather like knowing that your young brother will always be followed into the room by your father; once you've seen your brother come in, seeing your father follow him doesn't tell you anything you didn't already know, but you could have guessed with a 0.5 probability of being right. If however your brother could be followed by *anybody*, then there is no basis for guessing. Observing who follows him is much more informative. Such interdependence between successive data points is referred to as *serial dependency*.

Probability and Information

There is an exact relationship between the amount of information provided by an event and its probability of occurrence. Indeed this part of the definition of the unit of information, the *bit*, which is defined as that amount of information required to distinguish two otherwise equally likely options. Thus if I toss a coin and tell you the result, I give you one bit of information. If I toss it again, and give you the result again, I've given you two bits of information (note that the relationship here is logarithmic — two bits distinguishes between four option, three between eight and so on). The converse of this is that the more unlikely an event, the more information it contains. It follows therefore that being told something that was in any event predictable gives you little information; being told something you had no way of predicting gives you much more. If a series of pieces of information are related to each other in some form of sequence, the fact that each could have been predicted to some extent from the previous one reduces to a certain degree the information it contains.

What this means is that an item of data contains less information if it could have been predicted from previous items of data — or putting it another way, a set of completely independent data items contains much more information than a set where the items are to some extent correlated with each other. Unfortunately statistical tests like the t-test and the analysis of variance are unable to make allowance for the loss of information involved when data are not independent. They thus overestimate the amount of information contained in the data, and run the risk of drawing conclusions which are not justified. The outcome of all this is that such tests cannot be used unless the data points on which they are calculated are completely independent of each other.

When we conduct a study of a large sample of individuals, we randomly allocate each to either an experimental or a control group using each individual as a single data point. There is no reason to assume that the observations within each group are not independent. In a small-N study, however, there will often be reasons to expect some relationship between the successive observations, all of which will have been taken on a single individual. In a study of changes of heart rate, for example, we may find that our skill at taking pulse rates improves with practice as the experiment continues. Such increased skill may have no effect on the average measurement but a considerable effect on the error associated with any specific measurement, to the extent that the later measurements have less error than earlier ones.

It has been argued that where the data within a phase are generally stable, the successive data points *can* be regarded as independent. It has also been suggested that combining the data from the two A or B phases of an ABAB design will reduce the effect of dependency within observations since the error associated with (for example) the second A phase will be more closely correlated with that of the first B phase than the first A phase (Gentile, Roden and Klein 1972). In general however most researchers have been unconvinced by such arguments and have come to regard data which are serially dependent as unsuitable for conventional statistical tests.

Kazdin (1984) has suggested that the problem can be resolved by testing data for serial dependency using a procedure known as *autocorrelation*. In autocorrelation data are divided into two pairs, determined by a certain *lag* or delay in the sequence. Thus a list of data points like 2, 4, 5, 3, 6, 4, 3, 4, can be formed into a set of pairs by pairing each number with the next in the sequence (since there is no number following the last we end up with one fewer pairs than the original list of individual numbers). The list above could therefore be made into a set of seven pairs (from the original eight numbers) as follows; 2 4, 4 5, 5 3, 3 6, 6 6, 4 3, 3 4. Since each number is paired with the one immediately following it this is described as a lag of one. We could of course have a lag of two and pair each number with the next one but one — 2 5, 4 3, 5 6, 3 4, 6 3 (note that we now have only five pairs because both the last and penultimate number fail to have numbers following them with a lag of two). Such lists of pairs can be produced with greater and greater lags, each being paired with the one two placed behind it and so on. If these figures show serial dependency, that is to say if each number is to some extent correlated with the one which precedes it, then calculating a correlation coefficient on these pairs of numbers should reveal such interdependency. Indeed, a graph or *correlogram* can be plotted showing the value of the autocorrelation in the data plotted against the lag. For most serially dependent data the highest correlation will be obtained with a lag of one, with the correlation gradually decreasing as the lag increases; note however that where data show some cyclic variation a greater correlation may be obtained at higher lag values than some lower ones. Plotting the frequency of sunspots year by year, for example, shows the higher correlation at a lag of one (each succeeding year correlates most closely with the preceding one) but also a second peak at eleven years reflecting the cyclical nature of sunspot activity.

Kazdin (1984) argues that where calculation of autocorrelations fails to show any significant correlation then the data may be assumed not to be serially dependent and conventional t-tests and analysis of variance performed. Such a procedure is not however without its problems. First it should be noted that the testing of the significance of coefficients in a correlogram is not as simple as testing the significance of a single correlation coefficient; carried to its logical conclusion if the correlogram were calculated up to a lag of 100 the graph would be expected to contain five coefficients large enough to reach a .05 level of significance. Even where it is possible to calculate the significance of the correlogram data, it is important to remember that the failure to find a significant value does not show that the data are indeed independent; it merely shows that no interdependency has been found. Remember that a significant result shows that there is an effect, but a non-significant effect merely leaves the whole question open; it does not *prove* that there is no relationship. This is particularly problematic in the context of small-N designs where the number of data points is likely to be small and where in consequence the likelihood of detecting moderate amounts of serial dependency is lost. Under most circumstances, then, the use of tests designed for data which are not serially dependent should be discouraged with data from small-N designs.

An alternative approach is to use statistical tests explicitly designed for serially dependent data. Most prominent amongst such tests are those known as *time series analyses*. Time series analyses can be used with serially dependent data to detect the significance of such things as trends within phases, the significance of changes of level between phases, and other possible features of data gathered from a single subject. Time series designs take many forms and centre around the specification of particular models assumed to represent the processes generating the data. Unfortunately time series designs encounter exactly the same kinds of problem described with autocorrelations (indeed the calculation of a correlogram is the first stage of a time-series analysis). In particular, confident use of a time series design necessitates the gathering of large numbers of data points; Glass, Wilson and Gottman (1974) suggest that each phase of a study should include at least 50 data points. Experiments which collect few data points in each phase run the risk that meaningful effects will be regarded as non-significant simply because there is insufficient data to justify drawing the opposite conclusion. Put technically, the use of time-series designs with too few data points carries the serious risk of committing a type II error. It should be noted incidentally that time series designs are often intended for measuring the significance of change in data at a particular point (e.g. is there a significant change in the level of pulse between the baseline and experimental phases). In the kinds of analysis we have been describing (e.g. the ABAB design) it is important that the *totality* of the transitions be considered. That is to say, it is not enough to ask "could this particular change in level be due to chance?" but to ask "could each of these changes in level, occurring at these particular time, *all* be due to chance?" In this context careful specification of the time series model is necessitated.

It is not possible in this book to go into detail about how time-series analysis are conducted; such analyses merit a book in themselves. A good introduction to time-series analysis written from the viewpoint of the behavioural scientist is by Glass, Wilson and Gottman (1974). From the viewpoint of the small-N researcher, however, it seems likely that the time-series designs will be seen as appropriate for most of the types of study they are likely to conduct.

For multiple baseline designs, a simply nonparametric test R_n has been suggested as a means of testing the significance of changes when a treatment of experimental intervention is introduced. The principle of the test is that if treatment fails to produce a change in the behaviour the rank ordering of the results at each point of intervention will be randomly determined. The extent that the treatment makes a difference will be reflected in the ranks. Use of the test requires that the various multiple baselines be introduced in random order and that a minimum of four baselines be used (note that these could be either behaviours, individuals or settings).

The basic principle of the test can be illustrated with respect to the (hypothetical) data in table 5.2.

Table 5.2: Performance of four weightlifters before and after visualisation

Subjects	Training Sessions						
	1	2	3	4	5	6	7
1	58	64	61	63	65*a*	74	71
2	67	65	66	70*a*	75	72	69
3	65	60	67	61	65	70*a*	73
4	65	66	58	59	65	72	75*a*

In the table each of the four rows represents four different individuals in a weight training programme, and each of the seven columns represents successive training sessions. The figures in the table show the maximum weight in kilogrammes lifted on a particular exercise.

Imagine that the investigator wishes to investigate the potential benefit of teaching the athletes a visualisation technique to improve their performance. Use of R_n requires, as stated above, that baseline data be gathered on each subject and that the intervention be introduced on different occasions to each in a random sequence. The performance immediately following the teaching of visualisation is indicated in the table by the suffix *a*. Thus, the visualisation technique was first taught to athlete number 2, who learned it after the third training session; next it was taught to athlete number 1 who was taught after the fourth, then athlete number 3 after the fifth session and athlete 4 after the sixth.

Calculation of R_n is now straightforward. The first step is to take the column in which the first post-visualisation data occur — in this case, column 4 in which athlete number 2's first post-baseline performance is 70kg. The four individual performances are ranked and the position of the target athlete (number 2) is noted. In this case the individual in question has the best performance of the four athletes and obtains rank number 1.

The process is then repeated for the next column containing immediately post-visualisation data — column 1 which shows that athlete number 1's performance was 65kg. On this occasion the ranking is repeated but *only for the target individual and those still on baseline*. That is to say, individuals who have already had the visualisation before the current individual (number 1) are excluded. Thus, in the present example, the performances of athletes 1, 3, and 5 are ranked; all have the same performance and so all receive an equal rank of 2 (the average of 1, 2, and 3).

This process of ranking the individuals following any one person's experience of intervention continues until all have been taught the visualisation. Thus, in the table above, column 6 gives the post-visualisation performance for athlete number 3, and only this athlete and number 4 remain. Number 4's performance is better than number 3, so 3 obtains a rank of 2. Finally column seven has only athlete number 4 remaining, who of course thereby receives a rank of 1.

At this stage, then, we have the various rankings of the individuals immediately following the intervention when compared with those receiving no intervention. First was athlete number 2 with a rank of 1; then 1 with a rank of 2, 3 with a rank of 2 and 4 with a rank of 1. R_n is obtained simply by adding these numbers together, giving us 1+2+2+1=6. A table given by Revusky (1976) and reprinted by Kazdin (1984) indicates that a value of 6 fails to achieve statistical significance. To be significant at the .05 level (1-tailed) the ranks would in fact all have needed to be 1 — that is to say, with only four subjects all need to top their rankings for the result to be significant. As the number of subjects increases, statistically significant results can be obtained even if not all achieve top rankings once they have received the intervention.

The basic principle of R_n rests upon the notion that if the treatment is ineffective, then the individuals receiving the treatment should be no more likely to receive top ranking than any other individual. The table used to indicate significance is therefore simply a reflection of how far away any given result is from what would be expected from a particular sample size at random.

Effective use of R_n requires some degree of thought and caution. For example, in some situations it might not be expected that the intervention would produce its effect immediately; Kazdin (1984) suggests that under such situations several days or sessions should elapse between the introduction of the treatment with successive individuals, and the mean of the performances over these several days used for the rankings. Arguably such a procedure, where possible, is likely to produce more stable estimates than those based on a single performance. An alternative, where the effect of a treatment might be expected to be delayed, would be to specify *in advance* that the calculation of R_n was to be done on the performances an appropriate number of days following treatment. In doing so it is important that the number of days be selected carefully, that the same number of days be used for each individual, and that this be specified before the data are gathered. Thus the experimenter might believe that the treatment would take five days to become maximally effective. If so it might be appropriate to take for each individual the fifth performance following intervention and use this in the calculation.

Observant readers will also have noted that the technique becomes problematic when the baseline performances of the separate individuals is highly variable. For example, in the case of weightlifters it is unlikely that visualisation would ever bring the performance of a 50kg lifter above that of an 85kg lifter. Where the various baselines differ to any degree, the raw data used in the rankings should be replaced by an estimate (for each individual) of how much above or below their baseline data are the figures for the column under consideration. Indeed, for maximum sensitivity in the test it is preferable to use such a transformation even when baselines are broadly similar.

Acceptability Of Statistical Procedures In Small-N Research

By and large it is probably fair to say that the exponents of small-N research have largely ignored possible statistical applications to their research. Part of this is perhaps due to the context in which such designs have developed, that of applied behavioural psychology. This has generally proved extremely powerful, producing such large changes in behaviour that there has been little question that behaviour is different in baseline and experimental phases. Most of the effort in designing research strategies has been directed to increasing certainty that it is indeed the experimental manipulation which has made the difference (hence the range of possible designs such as ABAB and multiple baselines) and to determining the extent to which observations may be generalized (hence the variety of replication strategies). These are of course respectively issues of internal and external validity.

Advantages And Disadvantages Of Small-N Designs

Some of the advantages and disadvantages of small-N designs will by now have become apparent from the discussions in this chapter. The small-N design is less likely to be misled by the calculation of averages which bear no relation to any individual's performance. The small-N design may also have other advantages. It has been argued that the intensive study of a few individuals is at least as informative as the extensive study of a large number; the notion that it may be better to study one individual for a hundred hours as a hundred for one hour each. The small-N design has also been seen as having the benefit of increased flexibility. It is certainly the case that many small-N designs can be modified, as it were, in 'real time', the design changing in the light of the observations made during the early part of the experiment. Such changes are rarely possible in large group designs, where once the procedure has been used with a few subjects the same procedure will normally have to be maintained for the remainder. In principle the small-N design is also less limited than the large group design. Intrinsic to the statistical control of variability is a certain defeatism, which argues that no matter how much effort is made to track down and control variability a certain amount will remain which will need statistics to control. The small-N design, by contrast, argues that any factor causing a reasonable amount of variability in the data cannot be ignored as it is clearly part of the phenomenon. An understanding of the problem cannot be claimed whilst such sources remain unidentified.

At a more practical level, however the advantages of small-N designs are to a certain extent counterbalanced by practical problems. Perhaps the most obvious of these is the difficulty of obtaining sufficient control of sources of variability for many of the problems studied. In the field of human behaviour, for example, there may be a host of possible sources of variability in the data. Athletic performance for example may be moderated by both internal factors (e.g. motivation, state of health, level of training) and external factors (e.g. weather conditions, quality of opposition, availability of feedback). Obtaining sufficient control of each of these to reduce variability to a practical level may be difficult, and the researcher may feel obliged to turn to statistical rather than experimental control of such sources. On the other hand even this does not necessarily preclude the use of small-N designs, and a case can be made that the study of single subjects at a stroke eliminates many sources of variation (i.e. inter-subject variables).

In many situations the use of small-N procedures may not be possible because of the difficulty of gathering the requisite amount of data. An attempt to use the competitive performance of a marathon runner, for example, as a dependent variable would almost certainly be doomed to failure. Few competitive marathon runners run more than four or five such races per year, and many will run only one or two. On this basis it could take several years to gather sufficient data points to obtain a baseline, and even then this would probably be unstable as the athlete's performance changed naturally from year to year! It can, therefore, sometimes be necessary to choose dependent variables carefully, and certain variables may need to be ruled out completely.

Even when the data in question naturally occur with sufficient frequency, it may still not be possible to collect it. Observation of the rate at which individuals eat a plate of food is likely to be possible in principle, but is may take considerable determination on the part of the researcher, and a similar amount of patience on the part of the subject, if such data are to be gathered on a day-to-day basis. The use of small-N designs will almost always necessitate the collection of more data points per subject than extensive large group designs, and often this will imply greater demands on subjects' time. This can present major problems in subject recruitment, especially in the context of systematic replication where the researcher may be particularly in need of subjects with certain characteristics.

Besides the general problems of small-N designs there are also problems associated with specific procedures. We have already noted the possible problems of reversal designs, in particular that reversal may either be impossible (as when information has been imparted) or unethical (when a clinical benefit has been obtained). Multiple baselines may avoid these problems but then produce problems of their own. Within-subject multiple baselines, for example, require the experimenter to identify behaviours which will be independent but responsive to similar interventions - not always an easy task. Between-subject multiple baselines may present problems when the dependent variable is a function of important subject variables. This may result in one subject showing the effect but the next failing to do so (thus rendering the original multiple baseline an AB design with replication). Similarly changing criterion designs may have difficulty identifying with certainty the particular variable responsible for change. Requiring a judo player to defeat opponents of progressively greater skill may result in the player trying harder, and thus becoming fitter and stronger. Further improvement may then be a result of such improved physical condition rather than the teaching of a new technique.

It should also be noted that besides the scientific problems of small-N designs, there may also be problems of differing ideology between scientists. Whilst the scientific status of small-N designs is becoming increasingly accepted by researchers, it is still not uncommon to find experimenters brought up in the tradition of large-group statistical experiments who regard small-N designs as 'not real science'. Fortunately this appears to be less and less the case, and certainly professional journals, often reflecting prevailing scientific ideology, are increasingly publishing work reflecting the study of individuals which do not feel the need to have recourse to statistical testing (it is perhaps worth noting that the pages of *Nature*, one of the most prestigious of scientific journals, rarely involve statistical significance testing). Increasingly scientists are recognising that the issue is not one of a certain approach being superior to another but rather that certain designs have their own virtues. Certain problems will best be dealt with by large group statistical designs, others will be best dealt with by small-N designs, and for other problems both will have some strengths and weaknesses. It is perhaps important then not to think of small-N as being necessarily better or worse than large group designs in any absolute sense, but rather to acknowledge that under certain circumstances it may be the approach of choice whilst for other problems different methods may be preferable. Part of the skill of a competent researcher lies in devising methods of adapting research strategies to suit the problem in question. In this sense, the competent researcher is likely to need at least a basic awareness of what is achievable within a small-N framework.

Summary

1. Experiments with one or a few subjects - include the ABA, ABAB designs with simple extensions.

2. Selection of suitable independent and dependent variables, scheduling of experimental phases, systematic data gathering and display are all essential for small-N designs.

3. Multiple baseline designs are of particular value in applied behavioural psychology.

4. Special statistical procedures can be employed such as time series analysis and the calculation of R_n.

5. Small-N designs have certain practical problems such as the control of sources of variability, and the difficulty of obtaining the required quantity of data.

References

Barlow, D H and Hersen, M (1984) "Single Case Experimental Designs; strategies for studying behaviour change". Pergamon, New York.

Cooke, T P and Apolloni, T (1976) "Developing positive social-emotional behaviours; a study of training and generalisation effects". *Journal of Applied Behaviour Analysis* 9, 65-78.

Ferster, C B and Skinner, B F (1957) "Schedules of Reinforcement". Appleton Century Crofts, New York.

Gentile, J R, Roden, A H and Klein, R D (1972) "An analysis of variance model for the intrasubject replication design". *Journal of Applied Behaviour Analysis* 5, 193-198.

Glass, G V, Wilson, V L and Gottman J M (1974) "Design and analysis of time-series experiments". Associated University Press, Boulder, Colorado.

Hersen, M and Barlow, D H (1976) "Single Case Experimental Designs; strategies for studying behaviour change". 1st Edition, Pergamon, New York.

Kazdin, A E (1984) "Statistical analyses for single-case experimental designs" in D H Barlow and M Hersen (eds) "Single Case Experimental Designs: strategies for studying behaviour change". 2nd Edition, Pergamon, New York.

Revusky, S H (1976) "Some statistical treatments compatible with individual organism methodology". *Journal of Experimental Analysis of Behaviour*, 10, 319-330.

Sidman, M (1960) "Tactics of Scientific Research". Basic Books, New York.

Skinner, B F (1938) "The Behaviour of Organisms". Appleton-Century Crofts, New York.

CHAPTER 6

QUASI EXPERIMENTS

Key words : *double blind; confounding variables; matched subgroup analysis; analysis of covariance; multiple regression; cross-lagged correlation analysis; ecological validity.*

Introduction

We have seen how the random allocation to experimental and control groups enables the 'cancelling out' of variables other than the one(s) of interest. Thus if we wish to look at the effect of a particular training method, we randomly allocate the subjects either to an experimental group which receive the training method or to some appropriate control group.

Research questions often arise, however, in which random allocation to groups is not possible. If, for example, we are interested in looking at gender differences, we cannot randomly allocate our subjects to male and female groups; whether or not a subject is male is decided well in advance of our experiment!

Studies in which the experimental procedure does not permit random allocation to groups are known as 'Quasi-experimental' designs (Campbell and Stanley 1963). Such designs are common in the investigation of a number of 'real world' problems, as well as in some laboratory studies. Thus patients with a particular disease or injury might be compared with individuals who are healthy; crime rates in a city with one form of policing might be compared with crime rates in another with a different form; and athletes taking part in different events may be compared with each other.

Whilst random allocation of subjects to experimental and control groups might be seen as ideal, there may be a number of reasons why this cannot be done. The most obvious of these is that some allocations are simply not possible — as in the example of comparing male and female subjects. Even where random allocation is *in principle* possible, it may not be possible to do so *in practice*. Thus, in the example of the athletes given above, whilst one could in principle allocate athletes at random to, say, a sprint event or an endurance event, it is unlikely that the athletes themselves would be willing to accept such allocation. Moreover, such allocation would seriously threaten the realism of the study; in real-life athletes choose their own events. A study of athletes who had been 'allocated' to an event would bear little relation to reality.

Problems Of Random Allocation

When designing a study, there may be a number of factors which preclude random allocation of subjects to experimental and control groups. These include;

i. *Ethical issues*

Whilst allocation of subjects to one group or another may be possible, it may be unethical to do so. For example, it has been suggested that the use of strangulation procedures in judo might increase the risk of anoxic brain damage, caused by restriction of the blood supply to the brain. In principle this could be investigated by identifying a sample of judo players and allocating them at random to experimental or control groups. The experimental group could be given some kind of identifying marker which indicated that it was not permitted to use strangulation techniques on that person; the control group could be left to compete according to the usual rules. However such a procedure would give the experimental group an unfair advantage by 'protecting' them from a particular group of attacks from their opponents.

Such ethical problems constitute a major handicap in the investigation of the role of drugs like anabolic steroids in sport. From the point of view of a researcher, the ideal way to assess the benefits (if any) of the use of such drugs in competition would be to allocate athletes randomly to either a drug-taking group or a placebo group (i.e. a group who would be given an inert pill under the impression that it was the drug), with neither experimenter nor athlete knowing which group a subject was a member of (a *double-blind* study). Clearly however such a procedure would involve insuperable ethical problems, with the result that questions regarding the effects of drugs on performance remain difficult to answer.

ii. *Political issues*

Very often, although random allocation of subjects to groups might be defensible in terms of the ethical problems, it might still be impractical for political reasons. Thus, if a proposed new training method might be suspected of possibly causing as much harm as benefit, it would nevertheless be politically unacceptable to release details to only a random sample of coaches; if the method later turned out to be of benefit, those who had not been told of it would be resentful — and if it turned out to be harmful, those who had been informed would object! Either way, the body responsible for releasing information about training methods would be markedly unpopular.

iii. *Methodological issues*

Very often it may be the case that although one might be quite able, from an ethical or political viewpoint, to allocate subjects randomly to groups, nevertheless to do so would in itself invalidate the study. An example of this was given above, when we saw that allocating athletes to one event or another might be seen as ethically acceptable (since the athletes would take part in the study of their own accord) nevertheless this would be so unlike the way in which athletes normally come to choose their events that any results obtained would be completely unrealistic.

Confounding Variables

There may of course be other reasons which prevent the random allocation of subjects to groups — e.g. financial or practical reasons. Whatever the reasons, however, we are left with the problem that any subsequent comparison between the groups becomes more complicated than it would be with a conventional experiment. Any differences which are observed between two groups might not result from the criterion used to divide the sample into groups but from some other variable which *correlates* with this. We have already seen that it is impractical to have judo players randomly allocated to two groups, one of which is exposed to strangulations and the other not. Instead we might wish to investigate the role of strangulation by comparing a group of judo players who report having been frequently strangled with another which reports never or rarely having been strangled. Thus we might take a group of judo players, assess how often they had been strangled (this, of course, might not be so easy!) and distinguish between those who had been strangled frequently and those who had not. We might then administer tests of brain damage to both groups and see if the group who had been strangled frequently showed more signs.

Suppose that we do indeed find that the group which has been frequently strangled shows more signs of brain damage than the group which has not. Can we conclude that strangulation leads to brain damage? Certainly the data we have obtained are *consistent* with the theory that strangulation causes brain damage, but other explanations are possible. For example, it could be the case that judo players who are brain damaged when taking up the sport are less able to avoid situations where strangulation occurs. Judo is considered by many to be "the thinking person's martial art", and one could argue that competitors who are brain damaged would be less able to defend themselves than ones who are not. Thus, the finding that the frequently strangled competitors show more signs of brain damage than the infrequently might not indicate that strangulation caused brain damage, but rather that to be brain damaged results in a higher likelihood of strangulation. For example, it may be the case that being brain damaged makes a judo player less able to defend against being strangled — perhaps the brain damage makes it more difficult to see the attack coming, or maybe the damage impairs coordination preventing defence. In either of the latter two cases, we could find ourselves in a situation where individuals who were brain damaged before starting judo might be victims of strangulation techniques more often than individuals who were not brain damaged. Thus, after a period of time the brain damaged individuals would have been strangled more often than the non-brain damaged individuals, but it wouldn't be the strangulation which had caused the brain damage, but rather the brain damage which had caused the increased likelihood of strangulation.

The problem is of course one of difficulty in determining the direction of causality when two (or more) variables are observed to correlate. The fact that there is a correlation between brain damage and strangulation does not provide us with a single, definitive explanation. Strangulation could cause brain damage, *or* brain damage could cause an increase in strangulation, *or* both could be caused by some unknown third variable. For example, higher alcohol intake by some judo players might lead to increased likelihood of brain damage and decreased ability to defend against strangulation.

Clearly this is not an easy problem to solve, but it is not one which will simply go away if we ignore it. The kinds of questions asked in quasi-experimental designs are important questions, and if they can't be answered using a traditional experimental framework we have to make the best we can of the quasi-experimental methods. Because of this, quasi-experimental methodology has become increasingly sophisticated over the years. A number of advanced techniques being developed to help alleviate the interpretive problems which such designs involve. Although there isn't space to consider in detail the various procedures which have been developed in order to resolve the problems, a few general points can be noted. Perhaps the most important of these is the importance of identifying, and making allowance for, possible confounding variables.

For example, imagine that you have conducted a study looking at attitudes of two groups of sports people — say swimmers and sprinters. Suppose also that you find a number of differences in the attitudes of the two groups towards their sporting activity. All the problems we discussed in the context of the strangled judo players are repeated here. Are the swimmers and the sprinters different because there's something about the two sports which produce different attitudes? Or is it that swimming attracts people with one particular attitude and sprinting the other? Or are there simply some other differences between the two which might underlie the differences in attitudes?

Taking the latter question first, one initial step in trying to resolve the matter might be to see if there are in fact any obvious important differences between the two groups besides their chosen sport. For example, swimmers might be younger than sprinters — most competitive swimmers are in their teens, whilst many competitive sprinters are in their twenties or even older. If the mean ages of the two groups are indeed different, any differences in attitude might reflect nothing more than the differences in age rather than differences between the sports. Variables which vary between our two groups are known as *confounding* variables.

There are a number of ways to resolve this problem, but all basically revolve around the same general principle. An attempt is made to determine whether there is in fact a relationship between (in this case) attitude and the confounding variables. If we think for a moment, there are various simple ways we can check on this. The first, and most obvious, is perhaps to investigate whether or not there *is* a difference in age (or whatever) between the two groups. There could of course be a number of other possible differences between the two groups; for example, one group might contain a higher proportion of females, or the most prevalent social class background of the two groups might differ (a number of sports are more common amongst particular social groups — you might expect the average social background of three-day eventers or croquet players to be different from that of many soccer or rugby league players). One of the first tasks of the researcher using a quasi-experimental design is, even before any data are collected, to consider what factors might differ between the experimental and control groups and how they might affect the variables of interest. Thus, the researcher using a quasi-experimental design needs to gather data not only on the variables of interest but also on any possible confounding variables. For example, in the study of sprinters and swimmers mentioned above, we would wish to think about all the possible confounding variables which might affect our results. In gathering our data we would wish to record such things as age, sex, etc. Having gathered such data during the study, it is then important to scan the data and to check whether there are any obvious differences between the groups under study. This is in addition to that used to divide the sample in the first place — e.g. whether they are swimmers or sprinters. Commonly the data will be entered into a computer and t-test or analyses of variance or other calculations performed on the confounding variables. Using a computer it is quickly possible to perform such analyses before (or at the same time as) any attempt is made to analyse the variables of interest. If these analyses reveal that the groups differ significantly on any of the confounding variables this indicates the need for more careful consideration. As an aside here, it is worth noting that confounding variables which do not differ significantly may also need to be investigated further; remember that whilst finding a significant difference may justify our confidence that the two groups *do* differ, not finding a significant difference doesn't mean we can be confident that they *do not*. A good researcher will also look at the summary statistics (means etc.) and if they appear to be substantially different between the two groups will pursue the matter further even if the difference is not significant.

Clearly we cannot investigate *every* difference which might occur between the groups we are studying. It is likely that the groups differ in some ways we feel are likely to be important (e.g. age, sex) and others which we usually assume are not important (e.g. the colour of the walls of the room in which the data were gathered). Whether or not something seems likely to be important will depend to some extent on the particular study we are conducting. If we were measuring attitudes, for example, we might not be very concerned if one group were interviewed in the early morning and the other in the late evening. If however we were measuring their heights and weights this could be a critical confounding variable (we tend to be taller and lighter in the morning, shorter and heavier in the evening). It is not possible therefore to make a simple list of confounding variables which need to be assessed in all quasi-experimental designs. There are however certain variables which are so commonly likely to confound that they will normally be assessed as a matter of course. Examples of these are age, sex, social class, education and ethnic group.

In any particular study these variables will be supplemented by others relevant to the groups and the variables with which we are concerned. For example, in comparing two groups of sportspeople we may wish to take into account such factors as their level of ability at their particular sport (international, county, club, recreational etc).

Thus at the beginning of our study we need to determine as best we can (on the basis of theoretical considerations and existing literature) which potential confounding variables we need to examine. Once we have gathered our data we then compare our experimental and control groups on each of these variables and look for differences (remembering of course, as we discussed earlier, that failing to find a significant difference is not the same as proving that there *is not* a difference).

There are two possible outcomes of such analyses. Either the groups do differ with respect to one or more confounding variables, or they do not. The latter case is perhaps the simplest. If the confounding variables are the same in the experimental and control groups, then clearly they cannot account for any differences found between these groups. For example, if experimental and control groups have the same mean age, then differences between the groups cannot be explained away as an effect of age. Of course, it remains a possibility that the groups differ with respect to some other confounding variable that the experimenter has not considered. This is always a limitation of quasi-experimental designs. When using a pure experimental design, in which subjects are randomly allocated to experimental and control groups, it can be assumed that possible confounding variables will be equal in each of the groups. With a quasi-experimental design, in which subjects are allocated according to some pre-existing characteristic, there is always the possibility that some other factor, associated with this characteristic, is the one that lies behind our experimental differences.

Such problems are exacerbated when the investigator finds that the confounding variables *do* in fact differ between experimental and control groups. Such a finding places an immediate responsibility on experimenters to investigate whether the results could simply be ascribed to the differences in the confounding variables. For example, in the study we considered earlier of differences in attitude between swimmers and sprinters, we may have found on analysing our data that the sprinters were, on average, seven years older than the swimmers. Maybe it is just that older people have different attitudes to younger ones.

What we need to do under these circumstances is to determine the extent to which the differences in the groups are affected by the experimental and the confounding variables. The sophistication with which this is done will depend on a number of factors, including the expertise of the researcher, the characteristics of the data (in particular the sample sizes) and the state of existing research.

At the simplest level, it is possible to check whether or not the confounding variable could account for the differences by the simple act of checking the correlation between the confounding variables and the dependent or outcome variables. Remember that just because two variables correlate with each other, this doesn't mean that they correlate with a third. It is possible to have three variables, A B and C such that the correlation between A and B is 0.7, the correlation between B and C is also 0.7, but the correlation between A and C is zero. If the experimenter is lucky, there may be little or no correlation between the confounding variables and the outcome variables of interest. Such a situation is equivalent to one in which the confounding variables are the same in the experimental and control groups. In this case the variables are different, but they turn out to be irrelevant anyway. It is worth noting here that even when a confounding variable *does* turn out to be irrelevant, it was still worth measuring it. If it hadn't been measured, there would always have been some suspicion that this was the real reason behind any differences found.

At the end of all these analyses, the experimenter will commonly find that there do indeed remain some confounding variables which a) differ between experimental and control groups and b) do indeed correlate with the outcome variables of interest. Under these circumstances experimenters will usually perform supplementary analyses to clarify the possible role of the confounding variables in the results obtained.

Perhaps the simplest of such analysis is the *matched subgroup analysis*, in which subsamples are selected from the experimental and control groups in such a way as to match them according to the confounding variable. For example in a study in which the experimental group was on average three years older than the control groups, the researcher might take each member of the experimental group and try to find a member of the control group of similar age. If such a pair can be found, they are separated out and an attempt made to find a match for the second member of the experimental group. The process is continued until the experimental group has been divided into two; those subjects for whom an age-matched control can be found, and those for whom no such match is available. Taking the first set of subjects it is possible to repeat the original analyses knowing that this time the mean age of experimental and control groups will be the same. If the differences originally found between experimental and control groups remain when such matching has been done, then it is possible to conclude that some at least of the difference discovered cannot be accounted for simply in terms of age.

Such a procedure, although simple, is not without its problems. In the first place it is not always even possible; there may be too few individuals who can be matched in the two groups to make any statistical analysis possible. To some extent this can be overcome by relaxing the criteria for matching. Rather than being the same age, a match could be within one year, or two years, of the first individual. Carrying such relaxation too far may return us to the original problem if we then end up with groups of markedly different age. In general it is the case that the matched-subgroup method will result in some effective loss of sample size, with consequent loss of sensitivity of the statistical procedures used.

It may also be argued that in performing such matched subgroup analysis there is a consequent limit placed on the generalizability of the results. This is because the subgroups selected are inevitably a restricted range of the individuals under study. If, for example, it is very rare for swimmers to be in their thirties but not so rare for sprinters, only perhaps one or two of the sprinters (if any) will appear in the eventual subgroup. In consequence, older sprinters will be under-represented in the analysis. It may be argued that the subgroup analysis is only to check on the role of the confounding variables, and that the final conclusions should be based on the whole data set. However it is not impossible that the relationship between the confounding variables and the outcome variables may be different for older sprinters and younger ones. That is to say, in our present example, amongst younger sprinters age may make little difference, whereas amongst older sprinters it may be a significant confounding variable. Since our subgroup analysis would not check on this, it cannot be ruled out as a possibility.

Some of these problems can be minimized or avoided by the use of more complex statistical analyses, the details of which are beyond the scope of this introductory text. Amongst these are the *analysis of covariance* and the use of *multiple regression* techniques. The analysis of covariance, as its name suggests, is closely related to the analysis of variance, with the added characteristic that it aims to *partial out* the effects of the confounding variable. In our present example, the analysis of covariance can be thought of as a procedure which examines the data to determine the extent to which age and attitude are related and then applies a correction, based on this estimate, to the data to answer the question "what would we expect the difference to be if the groups *had* been similar ages?" Note that if a difference disappears when the effect of a confounding variable is partialled out, this does not necessarily mean that the experimental and outcome variable are not in fact related. For example, in a study of differences between attenders and non-attenders at a screening unit for breast cancer, Owens, Daly and Heron (1987) found significant differences in attitude. When the differences in age between the attenders and non-attenders were partialled out using analysis of covariance, the differences in attitudes disappeared. This does not however necessarily mean that there *is not* any difference in attitude; it may mean that older women are less likely to attend *because* of differences in attitude between older and younger women.

An alternative statistical approach to analysing quasi-experimental data is that of multiple regression. This is analagous to the use of simple correlations to predict one variable from another using a regression equation. The difference is that instead of trying to predict the outcome variable from a single experimental variable, a combination of experimental variables is used. In the procedure known as *stepwise* multiple regression, the increase in predictability of an outcome variable by successively adding extra experimental variables is estimated. Thus, in our example of attitude differences between swimmers and sprinters, we might first look at how well we could predict attitude simply on the basis of age (if age differed between the two groups) and then see if knowing both age and choice of sports produced a significant increase in our ability to predict. A finding that knowledge of sporting choice *did* increase our ability to predict attitude would be equivalent to saying that the attitudinal data could not be accounted for by age differences alone.

Such procedures do not exhaust the statistical armoury of the experienced quasi-experimental researcher. In particular, the use of correlational measures permits the testing out of particular theoretical models in a number of ways. For example, if a number of confounding variables are thought to interact in producing a particular outcome, study of the correlations between the variables permits statements regarding the various interactions. Such analyses are known as *'path analyses'*. In path analysis, a researcher may be interested in how several variables (for example neuroticism, maximum oxygen uptake, number of hours spent training) affect outcome (for example competitive performance). (S)he might have several models of how the variables might interact. The researcher might believe, for example, that whilst number of hours spent training affects maximal oxygen uptake, these two would be independent of neuroticism. According to such a model, performance would be the results of an independent combination of the maximal oxygen uptake (itself determined by number of hours training) and neuroticism. The researcher might however have an alternative model, according to which neuroticism itself is correlated with number of hours training — the more neurotic an athlete is, the more the athlete might feel driven to train. These alternative models would suggest quite difference patterns of intercorrelation between the variables. In the first model there should be a positive correlation between number of hours trained and maximal oxygen uptake, but little or no correlation between these variables and neuroticism. In the second model, by contrast, there should not only be correlations between number of hours trained and maximal oxygen uptake but also a correlation between neuroticism and number of hours trained. Analysing the patterns of correlations between variables in this way may help to clarify theories and in the construction of models.

Another way in which correlations might be used is in the procedure known as *"cross-lagged correlation analysis"*. In this the causal direction of correlational relationships can be clarified by taking measures of variables of interest at different times. Thus, to continue the example illustrated above, the experimenter might believe that excessive training might lead to neuroticism (rather than the other way around). In order to clarify this, it might be possible to gather data from each subject at the beginning and end of a specified time period (e.g. by taking two measures of each a year apart). If the correlation between neuroticism at time one and number of hours training at time two is greater than the correlation between number of hours training at time one and neuroticism at time two, it may be possible to conclude that it is the neuroticism which causes the increased training rather than vice versa. However this kind of cross-lagged correlation is considerably more complex in practice, and may be particularly sensitive to the statistical properties (e.g. the distributions) of the data. Again, this kind of analysis is usually best left to experienced researchers.

As mentioned earlier, the details of these procedures are beyond the scope of an introductory text. Such analyses are normally performed by advanced computer packages, and require, amongst other things, relatively large sample sizes. Where these are available, they provide a powerful means of increasing the sensitivity of quasi-experimental procedures.

Summary Of Steps In Conducting A Quasi-Experimental Study

i. Decide whether or not it is possible, practical and appropriate (e.g. in ethical terms) to allocate subjects randomly to groups. In particular ask yourself whether random allocation to groups would be so unpopular that only a minority of subjects would agree to take part. Ask yourself also whether such random allocation to groups would threaten the validity of the study by making it unrealistic. Remember that in a situation where people would normally make their own choice, random allocation may result in an unrealistic situation.

ii. If your answers to (i) above are such that you would be happy to conduct a study with random allocation to groups, this will normally be preferable to a quasi-experimental study. Otherwise you should be considering a quasi-experimental design. If this is the case, you should study the existing research literature and think carefully about the theoretical models relating to the phenomenon you are studying. On the basis of the literature and the theories make a list of possible controlling variables whose role in the final analysis you will wish to check.

iii. Gather data from your subjects, not only on the variables you are interested in but also on any possible confounding variables identified in (ii) above. It may be necessary at this stage to conduct a brief *pilot study* on a small sample to check that the data collection procedures are practical and acceptable to the subjects.

iv. Having gathered the data, calculate the means for the various confounding variables and identify any which seem to differ substantially between the experimental and control groups. For some variables other measures than the mean may be more appropriate. For example, for variables such as sex differences you may wish to use chi-squared or binomial tests.

v. If any of the confounding variables *do* appear to differ between the groups, investigate their role with respect to your outcome variables. At the very least you should consider procedures such as matched subgroup analysis, or the calculation of correlations between the variable you are studying and the confounding variables. Again, if you find that there is little or any relation between your confounding variable and the variable you are studying, your confidence in your results will be increased.

vi. If your confounding variables do indeed differ between groups, **and** they appear to be influencing your outcome variable, you may still be able to draw some conclusions from your study if the effects are still apparent in your matched subgroup analysis. If not, you may have to resort to more complex statistical analyses such as analysis of covariance.

Advantages And Disadvantages Of Quasi-Experimental Procedures

It would be a mistake to consider quasi-experimental designs in general as either superior or inferior to more conventional experimental designs involving random allocation of subject to groups. Under certain circumstances the use of a quasi-experimental design will not be as effective as a true experiment. In other circumstances the use of a true experiment may be such that the study would have to be highly artificial in order to fit the design.

For the most part quasi-experimental designs will permit studies of high *ecological validity*, that is to say ones in which the study procedure is highly naturalistic. Often a quasi-experimental study will involve little interference with existing routines. It should also be noted that quasi-experimental designs, as a result, may be no more difficult to interpret than true experimental studies. If for example we were trying to determine whether or not boxing is associated with brain injury, a true experimental design would either involve us in taking a sample of individuals from the general population and randomly allocating half to boxing lessons — meaning that a large number of people who would never dream of taking up boxing would be included — or of taking a sample of individuals interested in taking up boxing and randomly excluding half of them to act as a control group. Even the second option, which might seem a more reasonable option, would still be fraught with difficulties. For example, how might our control subjects react to being prevented from pursuing their interests? Would they go out and be involved in street fights instead? If so, any failure to find increased levels of brain damage in the boxing group might simply reflect that the damage acquired by the control group in their street fights was just as high as in boxing.

By contrast a quasi-experimental approach to the problem might involve a number of measures. A tough preliminary study might simply compare levels of brain damage in boxers with those in other competitive sports people of similar age, sex etc. If this showed higher levels of brain damage in the boxers, the next step might be to consider what other explanations, besides boxing as a cause, might be invoked. It might for example be argued that the drinking of alcohol is higher amongst the boxers than others; in this case a further study could be conducted in which alcohol levels were monitored, or in which schoolboy boxers below the age for drinking were assessed. Depending on the results of such studies, other possible explanations might be considered. If for example drinking levels were considered similar between the two adult groups, but the schoolboy boxers showed no higher likelihood of brain damage than non-boxers, these apparently conflicting results might provide a wealth of possibilities. If the children show similar levels of brain damage, this might argue that alcohol could be an important factor, but the failure to find differences in drinking levels might suggest that the effects of damage are less in childhood (is the brain still developing and able to compensate for damage) or that it is only after a number of years experience of boxing that the cumulative effects are apparent. Other possibilities might include differences in the social class background of groups compared; for example comparing boxers with tennis players might find a higher incidence of working-class origins in the former. Again, this could be checked by appropriate monitoring and careful analysis.

Looked at this way the use of quasi-experimental designs can be seen as an interactive process, each additional piece of information provided by a study suggesting possible interpretations, and challenging the researcher to design a further investigation or analysis to test out such interpretations. From this point of view, rather than being a ‘second best’ approach to research, the use of quasi-experimental methods can be seen as an exciting way of becoming intimately involved with the subject under study.

On the other hand, it cannot be denied that quasi-experimental designs inevitably leave open some questions about interpretation of results. Almost by definition, quasi-experimental procedures cannot unequivocally indicate the role of the variables under study. The downside of the exciting interaction between the researcher and problem is that there will almost always remain yet one more study to complete in order to rule out yet one more possible confounding variable. This is not to say that one cannot reach confident conclusions using these methods. For example, only a fool would question the link between cigarette smoking and lung cancer, even though the only studies demonstrating such a link in humans are quasi-experimental in nature. Often the use of a variety of research strategies can permit a problem to be clarified substantially without recourse to a randomised experiment. Consider for example an attempt to assess the relationship between injury rate and the provision of synthetic training surfaces in athletics. Injury rates amongst athletes could easily be monitored before and after the provision of a new running track, but there would always be the possibility that any difference observed before and after was actually the result of some other, unknown, simultaneous change (e.g. the screening of a TV series on injury prevention?) If however the same study were repeated every time a new running track were built throughout the country, then obtaining similar results each time would render it increasingly implausible that the difference could be attributed to anything else. With increasing number of studies, the number of confounding elements (e.g. screening of TV series) common to each occasion would be less and less. At a simple level the procedure is analagous to the method we use to determine whether a switch operates the room light; we press the switch and the room light comes on. If this happens just once, we might be willing to believe that it was coincidence, and that someone else pressed the *real* light switch at exactly the same time. If however the light consistently comes on each time we press the switch, we take only a few attempts to be persuaded.

Summary

There can be no doubt that the use of purely experimental designs, with random allocation of subjects to conditions, has had a major impact on diverse areas of research. Such procedures are however not without their problems. There may be practical difficulties associated with subjects dropping out of the study, and the procedure may need to be so distorted to fit the needs of the design that the results are hard to relate to the original problem of interest. When we add to these problems the possible political, ethical and practical issues it is apparent that such designs can only provide part of the researcher's armoury.

In the light of these considerations it is apparent that the use of quasi-experimental designs carried a number of advantages which may more than compensate for the interpretive difficulties involved. With carefully monitoring of the most likely confounding variables, and with skilled use of statistical analyses, quasi-experimental designs can often provide us with a means of investigating problems which would otherwise be totally intractable.

References

Campbell, D T and Stanley, J C (1963) "Experimental and quasi-experimental designs for research on teaching". in N L Gage (ed) "Handbook of Research on Teaching", Rand-McNally, Chicago.

Owens, R G, Daly, J and Heron, K (1987) "Psychological and social characteristics of attenders for breast screening". *Psychology and Health* 1, 303–313.

CHAPTER 7

ETHNOGRAPHIC STUDIES

Key words : *Qualitative vs. quantitative; non-participant and participant observation; reactivity; componential analysis; triangulation; internal validity; external validity; ethics.*

Introduction

A common complaint about much research is that the attempt to fit data collection into some kind of prearranged format means that the whole process becomes socially artificial. Such artificiality may be seen as a threat to the external validity of the data. The argument is that observations or information gathered in an artificial setting may reflect only behaviour specific to that setting. If, for example, we create a standardized test of an individual's behaviour, we might only obtain an artificial picture of that behaviour. If we specify particular questions to ask our subjects, we may obtain answers which only reflect ideas prompted by the questions. These may be specific, non-generalizable social responses rather than ideas or social activities which the subject might engage with 'naturally' using categories, vocabulary and social reference points on which they organise their everyday social lives.

In a recent study on inner city sport (Roberts and Brodie 1992), unstructured and semi-structured interviews were held with users of sports centres. This provided much information on attitudes and values which could not have been obtained by conventional structured interviews.

The style of research which has come to be known as *ethnography* makes particular and deliberate attempts to minimize artificiality in data collection.

Ethnographic research is characterised perhaps most strikingly by its attempts to study phenomena in as natural a setting as possible. Thus, only in the very loosest of senses might one think of an ethnographer conducting an experiment, and even then the 'experiment' might consist of nothing more than asking a respondent to speak freely about themselves or a phenomenon of interest.

Ethnographic research has been perhaps most widely used in sociology and social anthropology, although various kinds of ethnographic study have also been conducted in related subjects such as social psychology. The simplest form of ethnographic study is the interview. A central theme in ethnographic studies is the need to understand the socially-generated perceptions, motives and viewpoints of individuals. This can be done by giving individuals the opportunity to talk more freely than they can within artificial constraints of situations like experimental settings or by precisely-worded questions.

In conducting an interview, the ethnographer will therefore put considerable effort into giving the respondent (termed by some ethnographers the 'actor') as much control as possible over the conduct of the interview. Thus, an ethnographic interview might consist of little more than the interviewer asking the respondent to say something about themselves, or their work, or their community. Thereafter the ethnographer's contribution to the interview may typically consist of nothing more than noises of encouragement to keep the individual speaking.

Described like this, ethnographic research looks deceptively easy. In fact such research can be extremely difficult, both in conception and execution. Before commencing a study the ethnographer needs to put considerable thought into what questions might reasonably be answered by the research. It is then necessary to obtain suitable respondents, who are both willing to be approached and are likely to provide enough material to permit at least the development of initial ideas.

Typically the ethnographer doing such research will conduct more than one interview. Interviews may be audiotaped or even videotaped in order that the structure of the language and expression used may be more accurately recorded. However the use of such technology may be seen as in appropriate if it is likely to affect the results excessively. It could for example, inhibit the course of the discussion and thereby the flow of information. The interviews are often transcribed, analyzed and used to provide some degree of direction to future interviews by highlighting key categories or issues. In analyzing the data the researcher will be concerned with *qualitative* rather than *quantitative* aspects of the data. A particular issue may, for example, be given considerable attention because of its perceived importance rather than because of its frequency of occurrence. An issue which is important may crop up more often in the respondent's account than one which is trivial. On the other hand something may be referred to only once but appear to be central to the whole topic. Thus, a researcher conducting interviews with athletes may find that one makes reference to 'the friendliness of other competitors' or 'the opportunity to get to know people when the team have away matches'. Such comments may alert the researcher to issues of social contact and support in the sport. Another athlete may on the other hand concentrate on issues of the competitive potential. She may comment 'that's usually an easy championship to win' or 'the opposition is always tough at this event'. In this case the researcher may choose to investigate further such issues as performance relative to other athletes and the role of winning and losing. A third may appear to be particularly concerned with personal aspects of performance by stating 'that track is particularly fast' or 'you can always expect a strong wind on the back straight there, and times are never good'. Such an athlete might appear to be more concerned with personal achievement relative to previous performances, rather than relative to other athletes. Such issues might all be raised by a single athlete, some issues might be quite common amongst all athletes, whilst others appear to be idiosyncratic.

Ethnographic interviews were used with local authority leisure services officers to examine changes over time in recreation provision in inner cities. The following extract from Roberts and Brodie (1992) indicates how the interviews have been summarized.

> "However, by 1989 there were signs of change. Liverpool's design and development section was producing a detailed targeting policy in which groups would be prioritised. The two groups that had received most attention in practice were women and the unemployed. Liverpool had gone further than any other city that we studied towards formulating a structured programme for women. In 1986 the council had launched a "Women in Sport" campaign which ran for several years. In 1987 a policy document "Building Bridges" was produced by a Women and Sport Working Party which made recommendations on how to encourage women and girls to participate. This was accepted as departmental policy, and subsequently the council employed a Women's Sports Development Officer to co-ordinate provisions. The outcomes were an extensive programme of women-only activities at *all* centres, increased training for women staff, and an effort to change the image of sports centres which had appeared to promote male sports. Indeed, in each city activities popular with women such as aerobics and keep-fit, as well as more traditional sports such as netball, were being given more centre space and programme time."

The Use Of Observation

Probably the most widely known studies using ethnographic methods have been those which have involved direct observation of the individuals or organisations of interest. Such observation can take one of two forms, although it might be argued that these represent two extremes on a continuum. Observers may be external to the social setting (*non-participant observation*) or may actually become part of the system (*participant observation*).

Although non-participant observation is in many ways simpler than participant observation, it is not without its specific problems. Perhaps most obvious amongst these is the risk that being observed may actually change the usual behaviour of the individuals in question. Thus an observer studying children at play in a school playground might encounter the problem that the children spend a considerable amount of time attempting to engage the researcher. If this fails, the children may turn to discussing the question of why the observer is there. Clearly neither of these can be regarded as typical illustrations of the children's normal play behaviour, since neither would occur in the absence of the observer. This general problem of *reactivity* is a serious difficulty in conducting observations, and cannot always be overcome. Even the use of observation 'by remote control' e.g. by video or audio recording still encounters the same problem to a certain degree; the presence of the recorder may directly influence the behaviour of the respondent.

Of course it is not inevitable that the presence of an observer or a recording device will produce reactivity in the data. It is often the case that although there may be an initial reaction to the presence of the recorder, this disappears after a brief period of time. If the children in the above example failed to elicit any response from the observer, it would probably take only a fairly short time for the children to lose interest and return to their normal pattern of play. In a similar way, psychotherapists who have introduced audiotaping to their therapy sessions, and teachers who have introduced video and audio to their teaching sessions, have often remarked that it takes only a short time for those being recorded to 'forget' that the recorder is there and to return to the usual patterns of behaviour. However, two advantages of participant observation which are lost by non-participant observation are (i) the chance to improve the validity of the data by asking participants to talk about their actions and (ii) the chance to pursue social processes which continue 'out of frame'.

In most cases, though, whether recording behaviour through direct observation or through indirect means using recording devices, the researcher needs to be alert to the possibility that the observations being made are being affected by the very act of observing. At the same time it should not be assumed from the outset that such observation will necessarily lead to unsatisfactory or unrepresentative observation.

As with much ethnographic work, the researcher may need to turn to theoretical models or prior knowledge of such settings. This is to help determine whether and how the act of making observations will unduly affect the behaviour of those being observed. Perhaps the most obvious example where such observation might be expected to provide a sustained interference with natural patterns of behaviour is in the study of delinquent or deviant activities. Given that any objective record of delinquent activity could provide evidence against the perpetrator, and that being witness in such acts could lead to later testimony, it is unlikely that many offenders would behave in their usual manner when aware of being observed.

The ethnographer is therefore left with an apparently insoluble problem when it comes to the observation of deviant or criminal behaviour. Either an attempt can be made to observe the behaviour, in which case it will probably be inhibited and not occur, or it can be left to occur but observation will not be possible. One way round this is problem is to make the observations without the participants being aware that such observations are being made. This kind of procedure has been used to observe the patterns of interactions in clashes between rival gangs of football supporters, by means of remote video cameras. Such a procedure can of course only be used for observation at a distance, and is limited in the extent to which behaviour can be closely observed. It does not provide access to participants' own views or the categories used to explain their actions. In principle, however, the idea of making observations without the actors being observed provides a possible solution to the problem of reactivity. In an attempt to circumvent this kind of difficulty many ethnographers have turned to the second form of observation, that of participant observation.

In its purest sense, participant observation involves the researcher becoming a full member of the group, culture or society of interest. A number of ethnographic studies of this kind have been extremely widely publicised. In the United Kingdom for example, Patrick's (1973) study of a Glasgow gang is one of the best known. A social worker who looked considerably younger than he was, Patrick, managed to become accepted as a gang member by a Glasgow gang. His position as an accepted member of the gang provided him with a unique opportunity to investigate the activities, motivations and attitudes of gang members. Another dramatic example of the use of participant observation was conducted in the United Stated by Rosenhahn (1973), who with several colleagues succeeded in having himself admitted to a psychiatric hospital with a diagnosis of schizophrenia (the single researcher was admitted to a private, rather than a state hospital, was given a diagnosis of manic-depressive psychosis, a diagnosis with much better prognosis — despite the fact that all researchers had claimed identical symptoms when presenting!) In Rosenhahn's study the 'participant' status of the observers was in some ways unusual, in that having been admitted to hospital all researchers thereafter behaved quite normally; notably the staff of the hospital typically failed to notice that they were 'normal' (one researcher's taking of notes was recorded in the hospital as 'obsessional note-taking behaviour') whilst a number of the real patients recognised the researchers for what they were. Thus from the patients' point of view, Rosenhahn and his colleagues were outsiders, but from the viewpoint of the staff, who failed to recognise them, they were participants.

This variation in the extent to which a participant may become fully part of the system can be seen by considering other such studies. When Becker *et al.* (1961) for example carried out their participant observation study of medical students they did not attempt to pass themselves off as students, but nevertheless attended ward rounds, lectures, on-call duties etc. There was therefore no sense of their actually becoming medical students, and their identity and status were known to the individuals being observed. Thus, although Becker described the study as being a participant observation, it can be seen to be in many respects similar to non-participant observation. The distinction between the two approaches may indeed be one of degree.

Analysis Of Ethnographic Data

The data gathered in ethnographic studies can be analyzed in a variety of ways. Such analysis is itself dependent on how the data were obtained in the first place. Clearly the possibilities for analyzing verbatim transcripts of tape recorded interviews will be different from those appropriate to a long-term participant observation study. In this chapter we can only give a flavour of some of the methods which have been used. At the simplest level, analysis may consist of little more than a search of the content of interview data for significant or recurring themes or concepts. Even here however it should be noted that the skilled ethnographer will be alert to implied concepts as well as those explicitly stated. Consider for example, a comment like;

> "unemployment was a big issue even in those days; we were all out of work. One of the problems was that women took a lot of the jobs because of course it's cheaper to employ a woman.."

It may be that from the speaker's point of view, what is being discussed here is the problem of unemployment. However implicit also in the way the comment is phrased is a particular attitude towards the role of women in society. Comments like "...of course it's cheaper to employ a women.." hint at a belief that women's work is somehow less important, that women are not worth as much. This alone is not of course sufficient to indicate such an attitude with any certainty, as such a comment might be made by someone who felt that paying women less was unjust but nevertheless recognized that this was the way of things at the time in question. Note however the use of the phrase "... we were all out of work..." Since it has already been noted that *women* were perceived as having jobs, clearly women are not included in the use of the term 'we'. At the very least this seems to indicate that women are seen as separate, and might cue the ethnographer to return to discussion of the perceived role and status of women at a later stage of the research.

In may circumstances such qualitative analyses can be developed to a high level of sophistication. In the procedure known as *componential analysis* (Wallace 1972), an attempt is made to determine the structure of conceptual relationships for an individual or a community by determining the semantic relationships between terms used in describing such concepts. The procedure involved the following stages:

(1) gathering and defining terms used by the individual (note that such a definition should be from the individual's, not the researcher's point of view).

(2) determining the dimensions which underlie the terms (i.e. what makes the difference between an example of a term and a counter example).

(3) detailing interrelationships between such dimensions and

(4) from this deriving a statement of the relationships between the terms. In some circumstances it is possible not only to determine such relationships but also to identify levels of semantic and value ordering. Some dimensions, for example, are more important than others and carry implications for subordinate dimensions.

The use of componential analysis has been described by Taub and Leger (1980) in a study of the implicit taxonomy of individuals amongst members of a young gay community. Using this procedure they were able to identify dimensions such as sex and sexual orientation as important higher level dimensions, applying to all other dimensions identified. By contrast degree of overtness of homosexuality as a lower-level 'localised' dimension would apply only to some people, not others.

Whilst much data analysis in this field is of this qualitative nature, quantitative methods are also feasible. Linguists and anthropologists have devised a number of types of analysis whereby quantitative measures can be derived from data. Content analysis for example can involve the researcher in identifying particular words or phrases of interest. These are grouped according to similarity of differences in meaning (rather in the manner of the componential analysis described above). Measures such as the frequency or occurrence of such phrases, both in the text as a whole and possibly in conditional subsets of the text (e.g. how often is it mentioned in discussing topic A by contrast with discussing topic B?) can then be reported. The close involvement of ethnographers with their data gathering, particularly in participant observation, can be a considerable advantage. The researcher is able to use 'native categories' to 'make sense' of interactions and thereby guide the course of analysis.

Data analysis within ethnographic contexts is becoming increasingly sophisticated, as researchers use different means of making more and more use of the rich data such methods produce. A recent development has been the use of computerised methods to assist in data analysis. A computer program called *ETHNOGRAPH* for example can be run on a modest personal computer. It can provide considerable assistance to increase the speed of some operations in data analysis.

A final aspect of data analysis of importance to ethnographers is the concept of *triangulation* (Campbell and Fiske 1959). This refers to the use of several data sources to address the same question and provide further evidence of validity. For example, in examining a delinquent gang's involvement in criminal activities, the gang's own accounts might be compared and contrasted with accounts of victims, local crime rates etc. Such a procedure provides an opportunity for hypothesis testing within an ethnographic framework. Note that such triangulation need not be conducted entirely within an ethnographic perspective. Following Rosenhahn's study of psychiatric hospitals, for example he conducted a number of ingenious studies to test further the hypotheses generated. In one instance Rosenhahn noted that requests from patients for information were ignored, and it was hypothesised that this reflected the role of patients as perceived by staff. This was checked by later making other requests for information outside the hospital context. Even when the person approached was obviously in a hurry, the 'non-patient' was never ignored as he had been in the hospital. Perhaps more dramatically, to test out his hypothesis that grounds for detaining patients in hospital were somewhat arbitrary, Rosenhahn announced (following widespread publicity given to his original study) that further 'pseudopatients' were in other hospitals. In consequence the discharge rates from psychiatric hospitals rose, despite the fact that no such pseudopatients were in fact present. By drawing on additional sources and methods of investigation, it becomes possible to test the hypotheses generated during earlier stages of the study.

The basic stages in conducting an ethnographic study can therefore be summarised as follows;

i. Determine whether or not the questions to be addressed are appropriate to this particular kind of approach. Ethnographic studies are particularly suitable for studies which are attempting to discover how members of a particular group, organisation or activity see, make sense of and develop their own motives and reasons for acting.

ii. Decide on how the data are to be collected. For some purposes in-depth ethnographic interviews may be adequate. For other purposes some observation may be considered better. Observation (participant or non-participant) should be particularly considered if there is reason to believe that the attitudes or behaviour in question might be more generally socially unaccepted. Such problems might occur in studying deviant behaviour or socially censured attitudes (e.g. racism).

iii. Obtain access to the individuals or groups who are to be studied. Such access may be entirely straightforward or may be extremely difficult. For example, an ethnographer who is already a member of the group to be studied may have easy access to some sorts of information. Conversely to be an outsider breaking into a group, particularly one which has any reason to be defensive (e.g. oppressed minorities) may be extremely difficult. Note also that even an 'insider', acting in an unaccustomed way in order to gather information, may find that social barriers are put up. If possible, gather data from a number of sources in order to permit triangulation.

iv. Consider whether or when it might be useful to use more structured methods of data analysis, e.g. computerized analysis of field notes or content analysis of transcripts.

v. Write an account of the study highlighting social processes and categories you feel the study has shown and any implications of limitations on findings. Many ethnographers feel that it is appropriate to include in such a report a *reflexive account*. This describes their own feelings and responses whilst collecting the data and draws attention to how this might have influenced the observations make.

Strengths And Weaknesses Of Ethnographic Designs

For many people the greatest strength of ethnographic work is in its *internal validity*. By only providing the minimal level of interference with the system under study, there is considerable confidence that what is being studies is 'the real thing'. By contrast with what is seen as the artificiality of laboratory studies, ethnographic work is seen as highly naturalistic.

However such high levels of internal validity are not achieved without some sacrifice, in this case often involving considerable sacrifice of *external validity*. Typically an ethnographic study of a community or organisation will provide an extremely good account, rich in detail, but will often be difficult to extend to other organisations. To some extent this depends upon the range of data sources sampled. It is a little easier to generalise Rosenhahn's observations of psychiatric hospital (since several were involved) than Patrick's study of a Glasgow gang (of which only one was observed). The problem may be exacerbated by reliability concerns generated by the difficulty of replicating many ethnographic studies (e.g. few people would be in a position to gain admittance to a gang).

Discussion of the role of ethnographic work often leads to the suggestion that much of the strength and value of this kind of study lies in its ability to generate hypotheses and theories which can then be tested by other methods(e.g. experimentation, survey etc.) Certainly when it comes to the rigorous testing of a theory, ethnographic methods will rarely if ever permit unequivocal refutation. Even if the results obtained are unexpected, there will usually be scope for developing some kind of explanations of these results consistent with a particular theory. Unlike a laboratory experiment, where extraneous variables can be controlled to a sufficient degree to exclude their involvement in explaining away unexpected results, the range of imprecise data generated within an ethnographic study will usually permit a number of possible explanations. In this sense the ideas and hypotheses generated during ethnographic work may best be tested out through triangulation using other approaches (as in the Rosenhahn example described earlier).

Nevertheless, it would be a mistake to assume that ethnographic studies can never themselves be the site of hypothesis testing. In particular, ideas and hypotheses generated during the early stages of data collection can subsequently be explored in later stages. Most obviously this can be done directly, by asking respondents to clarify points that have been made earlier. Thus, in the example of the respondent discussing unemployment and women's jobs, it would be possible to ask the individual directly to say a little about how they see women fitting into the social group. The hypothesis that women are seen as separate would then be addressed directly. If the respondent talked of women as having a quite separate role this would support the hypothesis. Conversely a reply in terms of women's and men's roles being interchangeable would then probably lead to a request to clarify what was meant by the original comment.

An ethnographic approach provides a rich source of information with a high level of internal validity. This information is suitable for analysis in a variety of ways. These can both provide hypotheses for further testing and to a certain degree their actual testing. The hypotheses generated can also be tested using other approaches, as for example when a small intensive ethnographic study forms the basis for a questionnaire used in a large-scale survey. In addition to specific hypothesis generation, ethnographic data can also indicate the way in which people use a range of alternative categories and accounts to make sense of their actions.

A further advantage of the ethnographic approach is its flexibility. Unlike a large-scale survey, or some tightly controlled laboratory experiments, the type of data gathered during an ethnographic study can have a substantial influence on the subsequent development of later or related research. Ideas generated from the early part of the data gathering can be further investigated directly during the later stages of the study. Again, this relates to the particular strength of the ethnographic approach as a means of generating (and sometimes testing) hypotheses.

The disadvantages of the ethnographic approach are that the external validity can be compromised, in particular by the limited range of subject matter which can usually be accessed in the time available. There is also a degree to which such studies are necessarily influenced by the expectations, biases and prejudices of the investigator. It is to be hoped that the good ethnographer will minimise the extent to which this occurs and that the inclusion of a reflexive account in the final report will enable readers to judge for themselves the areas and effects of such bias.

We have seen that the very act of being observed may influence the behaviour of the respondents, and the way in which methods such as participant observation can be used to avoid this. The use of participant observation has its own specific problems. For a start there may be serious practical problems. In Rosenhahn's study, even when the investigators were behaving normally, there was considerable reluctance on the part of the hospital staff to discharge them as 'normal'. Typically when the investigators did manage to be discharged it was not as 'cured' but as 'schizophrenia in remission'. Patrick found that as a member of a Glasgow gang, the behaviour expected of him took him close to the boundary of what would be illegal. These and similar problems mean that covert participant observation should not be undertaken without careful thought. The extent to which the researcher is prepared to trade personal patterns of 'normal' behaviour and values for the purposes of research has to be considered carefully.

It can be argued that the philosophical stance from which an ethnographic perspective is derived is not as secure as it might appear. Psychologists in particular, ranging from the psychoanalytic to the behavioural, have commonly noted that people may act without being aware of the reasons for doing so. Often people may give reasons for their behaviour which are uninformative. "I did it because I felt like it.." is the kind of comment which seems plausible to many but which begs the question of why the individual "felt like it". At times the ability of the individual to identify their own motives may be questioned. When asked to explain the motive for teasing a loved one, the respondent may sincerely believe that it is to amuse them. A Freudian, however, might wish to invoke an explanation in terms of symbolic aggression. In many circumstances the individual may actually have no explanation at all for their own behaviour. This may be seen for example when an individual is engaged in some form of self-destructive behaviour like self-cutting or bulimia and then says to a therapist "I can't understand why I do it."

Certainly most ethnographers would concede that simply asking why someone does something and then expecting the immediate reply to provide 'cause' or 'motive' as a complete explanation is inadequate. To suggest that this is the essence of ethnography is however to caricature unfairly the reality of the approach. In identifying the motives, viewpoints and vocabularies of respondents, the ethnographer will often gain clues. To go beyond the surface presentation of an account and look for implied meanings, interrelationships between concepts and sequencing of natural processes and meanings can give rise to a variety of understandings considerably more sophisticated than the caricature would suggest. Moveover, it has been suggested that even when an individual's expressed reasons do not tell the whole story, they still cannot be ignored. If a person believes that a particular motive underlies their behaviour, that belief itself needs to be considered.

Ethical Implications

It is appropriate here to remark that the use of certain ethnographic procedures, most notably covert participant observation, may raise serious ethical problems. If we consider Patrick's study of gang behaviour, it could be argued that by deceiving the gang into believing he was 'one of them' in the sense of holding common aims and priorities he was acting unethically. Certainly it would constitute an example of involving someone in a research process without their permission. This is a course of action which would normally require extremely persuasive arguments to justify. The enthusiasm the gang appeared to have for seeing themselves written about in the press argues that they would have approved wholeheartedly. At one level such a study can be seen as little more than spying on a group. If one were to suggest such spying on groups with a higher social status and power, (e.g. a study on nurses without their permission) there would be an outcry around the issues of the rights of such groups to own information about themselves and to control the circumstances of its disclosure. Yet if spying on groups viewed positively by society is unacceptable, it can be argued that the same objections apply to obtaining and disclosing information about a group viewed negatively.

Such a difficulty is illustrated well by another participant observation study, (Humphreys 1970) in which the researcher investigated casual homosexual encounters in public lavatories in the U S A. By passing himself off as a voyeur, interested in watching the sexual behaviour of others, he was able to obtain a considerable amount of information about the patterns of such encounters. Amongst the details given in his final report are accounts of the characteristics of the kinds of public toilets in which such behaviour takes place. It is not difficult to see how publication of this information might lead to increased effectiveness of policing and thereby increased persecution of a minority group. The use of such covert participant observation to benefit a researcher's aims to the detriment of the group observed can therefore be seen to be taking the researcher onto very dubious ethical ground. Even where the consequences of being observed in this way are less serious than in the Humphreys example, there are general principles of privacy and entitlement to refuse to take part in research to be considered. It is difficult to see how such principles can be observed in this kind of study, and it can be argued that overriding of such principles should require a strong justification.

In some circumstances the ethical problems of covert observation can be ameliorated to a certain degree. At the very least this is likely to involve a thorough debriefing of participants once the research is complete, with an opportunity to veto the information that has been gathered. An additional safeguard might, with some participants, actually involve them being given permission to veto any part of the final report to which exception is taken. In practice however such courses of action will rarely be open. Returning to a violent gang to explain that one is not, after all, a friend but is instead a spy might have fatal consequences. In the case of the Humphreys study of casual homosexual encounters, it is unlikely that many of the participants could actually be traced. Indeed it could be argued that publishing the kind of information put at risk individuals who were not part of the original study. In many circumstances the problem of constructing a 'final report' in non-academic's terms may make informed consent very difficult.

Summary

Ethnographic approaches to research provide a means of obtaining rich sources of information which centre on the *individual's* own psychological processes underlying actions and the social processes which structure them. Although such approaches can appear simple at first glance, they will usually involve extensive skill in balancing many qualitative considerations at all stages — design, execution and analysis. In particular the researcher will need to give careful thought to the extent to which conducting a study will itself influence the behaviour of the individuals concerned. Whilst varying degrees of covert observation (participant and non-participant) may help circumvent problems of reactivity, they throw up their own practical and ethical problems. Nevertheless the increasing sophistication of execution and analysis of ethnographic studies points to a substantial role for these methods in increasing the understanding of social systems and in generating and testing of specific hypotheses. Triangulation with other approaches substantially increased their validity, and it seems likely that in future researchers will need at least a basic understanding of the approach.

References

Becker, H S, Blanche, G, Everett, C H, and Anselm, L S (1961) "Boys in White: student culture in medical school. University of Chicago Press, Chicago.

Campbell, D T and Fiske, D W (1959) "Convergent and discriminant validation by the multitrait multimethod matrix". *Psychological Bulletin* 56, 81-105.

Humphreys, L (1970) "The Tearoom Trade". Duckworth, London.

Patrick, J (1973) "A Glasgow Gang Observed". Eyre Methuen, London.

Roberts, K and Brodie, D A (1992) "Inner-City Sport: who plays, and what are the benefits". Giordano Bruno, Culemborg, the Netherlands.

Rosenhahn, D (1973) "On being sane in insane places". *Science* 179, 250–258.

Taub, D and Leger, R (1980) "'Drag queens' and 'Fag hags': two social identities and a gay community" in R F Lawson and R Knapp (eds) "The Sociological View". Oxford University Press, Headington, Oxford.

Wallace, A F C (1972) "Culture and Cognition" by J Spradley (ed). Chandler, New York pp. 111–126.

CHAPTER 8

SURVEYS

Key words : *pilot study; information content; sampling - simple random; systematic; stratified; cluster; stage; volunteers; survey panels; planned observations.*

Introduction

Survey designs are commonly used in human movement and health sciences to:

(i) establish the characteristics of a community of population

(ii) provide background data for intervention

(iii) observe changes over time

(iv) predict the outcome of an event in which the population surveyed are involved.

The characteristics of a community can be surveyed from hospital records, (e.g. heart disease per head of population) from dental records, from doctors' notes, from population censuses, from household surveys and many other sources. The information can be used as a comparison with other groups as shown in Table 8.1.

Table 8.1 Heart disease rates on Merseyside

	Death Rate per 100,000			
	MEN		WOMEN	
	Crude	Age Adjusted	Crude	Age Adjusted
Chester	335.9	349.1	245.2	267.1
Crewe	360.4	374.9	297.2	325.9
Halton	335.8	408.5	248.7	320.9
Liverpool	387.1	390.0	328.4	304.2
Macclesfield	300.3	295.2	251.6	257.2
Southport and Formby	417.3	363.3	398.1	294.0
South Sefton	356.9	376.4	267.6	279.0
St Helens and Knowsley	343.7	398.3	238.8	286.1
Warrington	329.5	380.8	291.0	342.0
Wirral	365.0	354.6	297.1	274.7

Background data before intervention is another valuable application of surveys. For example, a physiotherapy department may wish to introduce spinal manipulation as a treatment modality. The benefits of this new form of treatment (intervention) are best assessed against a background of information from before the intervention is introduced. Therefore careful records of cases presenting, treatment time, and recovery rates would be surveyed before the intervention is employed. Only on this basis will the efficacy of the treatment be known.

A survey to monitor changes observed over time could be exemplified by hospital records of low birthweight babies. It could be hypothesized that increased unwanted pregnancies, in combination with a higher incidence of female smokers will result in a greater number of low birthweight babies. Surveys of birth weights every five years over a 30 year period will provide evidence for the hypothesis if other variables (smoking levels, unwanted pregnancies, dietary improvement) can either be measured or controlled.

A survey to monitor the impact of AIDS awareness advertizing on television could be used to predict the outcome. It could by hypothesized that if the commercials were aimed at teenagers and shown at times when teenagers tend to watch television that they would show the greatest change in awareness. A survey on the topic to provide AIDS awareness values for all viewers irrespective of age would provide an initial baseline. Immediately after the advertizing the same population could be re-surveyed and the prediction evaluated.

Planning The Survey

The first stage in planning a survey is to establish a clear *statement of the problem*. Often the enthusiasm to undertake the survey obscures what underlying problem requires the information. In the health and movement sciences the problem could be associated with changes in health care, introduction of new management systems, the evaluation of a specific campaign, establishing levels of fitness in a community or current knowledge, perceptions or awareness. The researchers may only be interested in obtaining 'benchmark' data to make comparisons at a later stage. They may, however, be more concerned with relationships between variables. The sponsors of the survey may consider that respondents from different geographical areas, ethnic groups or social classes have different levels of health, fitness, sports participation or immunisation and wish to test these assumptions.

It is essential that the general nature of a problem is converted into a clear definition that can be examined objectively. This process of *delimitation* will prevent 'trawling' research surveys where a wide range of questions are asked, many of which become redundant. It is often valuable after the first draft of the questionnaire is produced to have a group discussion to decide which questions are absolutely essential to fulfil the *purposes* of the research.

At the same time, the potential *consumer* of the research should be considered as a guide in the final decisions on the inclusion or exclusion of questions.

Increasingly survey work in the health and movement sciences considers public opinion in addition to questions of fact. It is essential to recognize the impact of timing on public opinion surveys. A health-related topic could easily be influenced by a television broadcast the previous evening or a campaign by a local paper. In some cases, of course, the survey has been designed to establish the impact of a campaign, but the recognition of extraneous influences is essential. The publication of public opinion issues must also be rapid if it is to be meaningful to the consumer. There is limited value in seeking the views on a recent outbreak of legionnaire's disease if by the time the survey is published the source of the problem has been identified and eradicated.

It is necessary to establish whether a survey is the appropriate method to obtain the required information. One public health issue, for example, may be poor housing. A survey which reveals that inadequate housing is evident in 25% of the population would have far less impact than a documentary on the living conditions of the poorest sector of the community.

The eventual consumer of the survey can have a greater or lesser involvement in its production. Awareness of the consumer may prevent the results being misinterpreted at a later stage.

Surveys which study the impact of a particular innovation (e.g. building a new sports centre on participation) may be totally ineffective because of a lack of information from before the event. Human memory can be unreliable so it is essential to resist surveys which cannot provide the required information. This also emphasises the necessity in any evaluative work to obtain the baseline data before the intervention occurs.

In planning a survey it is necessary to ensure that the results will get to the client or consumer before the material becomes dated. If the survey is to be the basis of action then it may have to fit into expenditure schedules. Typically the fiscal year is different from the academic year. This also applies in funding surveys when the money may come available in April which is not a good time to recruit staff.

The overall level of finance is essential information in planning survey work. As it will most often involve trained personnel, working anti-social hours over relatively long periods of time, the procedure can become expensive. Even if using student labour to gather the data, such aspects as travelling expenses, printing the questionnaires and data processing have to be costed properly. It is quite common to undertake a pilot study which will provide a good guide to the costs of a full-scale survey.

Other resources to support the survey must be known in advance. Crucial to this is the project director who may have to make on-going decisions about the phases of the project. A testing programme on aspects of health and fitness could be seriously prejudiced as a result of industrial action. A delay of only 2–3 weeks in an early phase of the work could easily have repercussions if later phases of the survey were designed to fit around annual holidays. It is not uncommon for factors not initially recognized, or not within the control of the researchers, to require changes of survey strategy. In such cases, a full knowledge of available resources would be essential.

There are many instances when it is desirable to use the resources of a professional research agency. If speed is important, a commercial organization is more likely to have trained staff already in the field. It is also possible that a survey with few questions could be added to one that is about to be undertaken for another client and thus eliminate the need for a separate survey. It is important when employing a commercial organization that a detailed brief is provided. They will only quote a price for what has been specified. One cannot assume that additional work which may be expected of students who have different motives, will be undertaken without renegotiation of the fee.

Another feature of planning is to be confident that the answer to the questions is not already known. A literature search would clearly be a prerequisite of any survey but the sources held on literature retrieval sources may not always be complete. For example a question on the incidence of cigarette smoking may be a legitimate question in a local survey for which values are not known. A subsidiary question on brand of cigarette smoked may be difficult to locate in a literature search, but may be known to the manufacturers who could provide the required data. Information which has been published may have been presented in a manner which is inappropriate to the survey currently being planned. However a reorganisation of the data, perhaps presenting the raw material differently could save a lot of unnecessary work. One needs to be cautious because using data from previous work runs the risk of being dated and may not apply to changed circumstances. An example of the latter would be boundary changes which re-define geographical areas.

The method of collecting the data has to be considered once the problem has been clearly formulated. This requires familiarity with the options available and a recognition of the strengths and weaknesses of different approaches. If a particular method does have disadvantages, the researcher may have to consider methods of getting around them.

Inexperienced researchers should recognize their limitations and be prepared to consult with more highly trained specialists. If the survey is important or extensive it would be desirable to have a group of advisors, especially in the initial stages. Particularly seek advice from people who have surveyed the locality previously. It may be desirable, for example, to consult with local community groups to obtain the best response rate and this may not be recognized without local advice.

Deciding On The Survey Type

Surveys most commonly ask a series of questions to a large group of people. However surveys can be a single question e.g. "Which candidate did you vote for?" in an exit poll at a by-election, or can involve a measurement e.g. cholesterol levels in an 'at risk' population.

At the same time as the individual questions are being formulated it is essential to establish how the questions are to be asked. If it is to be a postal survey there will be no researcher on hand to explain difficult questions. More importantly no one will be available to check that all questions have been completed. The presence of an interviewer overcomes these difficulties but may be considered intrusive, will reduce the element of confidentiality and is more costly. On balance the availability of the interviewer is desirable because the scope and style of the questions can be more varied, open or closed questions can be used, prompting becomes feasible and a non-structured approach is possible.

Designing The Survey

The pilot study

This is the opportunity to examine the design of the survey so that when the survey is undertaken in its entirety all the design issues will have been clarified.

The subject, the response rate, the ease of answering the questionnaire, the time taken, the technique of collection, and the problems of a given locality can all be pre-tested. It is a common fault to assume that the reaction, understanding and knowledge of the researcher is similar to the person to be surveyed. It may be necessary to test a survey procedure in distinct areas to gauge different responses. A socially deprived area may have difficulties in comprehension whereas a socially advantaged area may be suspicious of strangers. Two techniques may need to be trialled and will need a comparable sample to examine which method is best. Eliciting suitable information on ethnicity, salary, employment and socio-economic grouping can be achieved in a number of ways, and the pilot study gives the opportunity to establish the best approach.

The use of a self-completion questionnaire requires a very thorough pre-test to ensure that the questions are understood and answered as the researcher intends. This is especially the case if the respondent is to miss out certain questions as a result of a previous response. If this is not clear, the respondent can become not only confused but annoyed at what appear to be redundant questions and may fail to complete the questionnaire as confidence in it is lost. It is well worth drafting questions, showing them to colleagues for initial criticism, pre-testing them on the extremes of the likely respondents (oldest, youngest, least educated, most antagonistic) and reviewing and revising them before the survey is started. It must be remembered that the researchers who undertake the survey may not personally be interested in the findings of the questions and are simply employees. A problem in which you have great enthusiasm may be treated totally objectively by others.

Ideally pre-tests should be undertaken on a different, though similar group from those to be examined in the full survey. This prevents contamination of the final results by respondents already appraised of the content by being involved in the pilot survey. It is of no value piloting a questionnaire on a convenient group such as students because they may be totally unrepresentative of the intended population.

The size of the pilot study will depend on the extent of likely revisions. If the questionnaire is straightforward, less than 100 respondents may be sufficient. With a more complicated survey, when the procedure itself is being examined, more respondents will be required. A much lower number (e.g. 25) may be sufficient if a simple choice of two ways to put a single question is all that is being examined.

Occasionally a pilot study requires no modification to the questions and in that case it is acceptable to incorporate the pilot into the main study provided the time between the two is acceptable.

Finances

Most surveys operate on a limited budget which will often control the detail that can be examined. Low budget surveys may lead to less questions being asked or less highly qualified employees or less computer time being available for the data analysis. In the case of a single research worker undertaking a minor survey with no additional resources the financial budget effectively becomes a time budget. The main subdivisions of cost will include the planning stage, the investigative phase and the data analysis phase. As a starting point it may be useful to consider these phases as requiring one third of the budget each and then justifying any variation from this division of expense.

All possible expenses should be itemized in the knowledge that any reduction in available funds will result in certain items being re-costed. This may have further implications for other items of expenditure and planning. If, for example, funds were not available for travelling expenses for a student-based survey, it may be necessary to select students that live in the locality of the survey.

When planning surveys which take longer than one year, or longitudinal surveys which are repeated annually, the costs attributed to inflation, salary increments and pay awards need to be planned into a cumulative budget.

Time

A detailed schedule for each phase of the work should be prepared to show the starting and finishing points. A time estimate blank similar to the critical path analysis blank in Chapter 11 should be used which shows which phases are sequential and which are running in parallel. All sorts of reasons prevent a complex survey keeping to time. These include sickness and absenteeism, holidays, equipment failures, misunderstandings, orders not being received etc. Some cannot be predicted in advance but recognition is needed that tight time schedules are difficult to maintain. It is quite clear that certain surveys involve a rapid response and publication. These would be illustrated by exit polls at by-elections. However most surveys of any substance in the area of health and movement science will take several months from data collection to publication, especially if the analysis is being undertaken ‘in house’.

The time of year to conduct a survey will introduce certain variables. The summer holiday period is best avoided because many respondents will be away and those who do not go away may be an unrepresentative income group. Religious holidays are also unrepresentative times because people often travel to be with family members and will not be at their normal residence. The time of the week is another variable with weekends having a different eating, activity, work and social profile for most people. Nutritional and physical activity surveys often examine one typical week day and one weekend day to try to obtain a better balance.

Limiting the range of the survey

A common fault in survey design is using the opportunity for unrestricted questioning. This temptation should be avoided because although it may appear an opportunity lost, it often results in an unmanageable questionnaire and redundant information.

A recent survey on indoor sports could have surveyed over 40 different activities, but such a survey would have been too large to manage within the resources available. Thus a decision was made to survey *representative* sports which included:

(i) a large age range

(ii) both males and females

(iii) a wide socio-economic and ethnic mix

(iv) energetic and non-energetic sports.

It was also desirable to take into account other external factors such as the policy of the Government or Sports Council with respect to the sports under selection. Thus from the initial list of over 40 options, the final selection of seven sports was indoor soccer, badminton, swimming, keep fit/aerobics/weight training, snooker, bowls and martial arts. Seven indoor sports seemed a reasonable compromise between the range available and having a sufficiently small number for the sample sizes to be large enough for valid comparisons.

Information content of the questions

It is a common error to include questions which do not produce useful material. The nature of questionnaires is that including a few additional questions may not on the face of it produce problems. Unlike a laboratory experiment where adding further tests will be very time consuming, this is likely to be marginal with a questionnaire. However this fails to recognize the perceptions of the respondents who must see the relevance of the questions. It also fails to recognize the additional processing time (and cost) of additional questions when the information content may be marginal.

Example

A survey on cigarette smoking asked the reasonable question "How many cigarettes do you smoke per day?" and provided a box for the answer. A subsidiary question was "What brand of cigarettes do you smoke?" and provided a space for the answer. The latter question clearly provides information on manufacturer, tar content and if related to current advertising, would give an indication of marketing impact. If the researcher specifically wished to gauge the manufacturers' proportion of the market or the influence of high tar cigarettes then knowledge of brand is useful. However the brand proportionality within the population will be available from other sources (albeit often the manufacturers themselves who may provide distorted information). The tar content will be a direct extrapolation from the brand and numbers smoked. In this particular example the question on brand was deliberately asked in a local survey to establish the perceived damage by a given manufacturer in a specified city and was thus justified. If the survey had been a nationwide one, the justification for the question would have been far less.

The individual questions need to be considered carefully in relation to the original hypotheses for the overall survey. It is far better to exclude an individual question if there is insufficient confidence that it will produce worthwhile information at the completion of the survey.

Obtaining The Information

This can take the following forms:

The direct interview
Planned observation
Recorders
Radio and television
Telephone interviews
Postal questionnaire
Survey panels

1. The direct interview

This technique is likely to produce the most detailed response because human judgement can be used to ensure the appropriate outcome. If, for example, a designated respondent in a household is intended, the interviewer can judge whether another person can answer the questions if the door is not answered by the correct person.

As long as the interviewer is diligent in finding the respondent, which may mean repeated calls or interviewing at his/her place of work, a very high percentage of acceptable returns can be achieved.

Most commonly the interviewer will introduce him/herself and use a prepared questionnaire to guide the survey questions. For quantitative analysis a very rigorous questionnaire will be used, but even the best may not be fully understood by the respondent. The advantage of the direct interview is that any uncertainties can be answered and the respondent can be assisted to understand the questions fully.

The direct interview has an additional benefit of being able to use observation to establish personal characteristics. It may be necessary, for example, to obtain an inventory of all living-room equipment in the home as used in Chaplin's Social Status Scale. For reliable recording it would not be possible to rely on a self-completion questionnaire but for the interviewer to be present in the house.

Similarly if any physical measures were required, even as simple as height and weight, the direct interview is ideal because self completion reports of height and weight are known to be inaccurate, with weight consistently under-reported.

The direct interview is most usual when a reaction is required to visual information. This is most commonly used when responding to market research on brands but can be used with effect in the health sciences. For example a recent survey on the public's attitude to sponsorship of smoking required a response to a series of advertisements which were shown to the respondents.

Similarly there are occasions when responses may have to be sorted into piles (e.g. recreational activities into daily, weekly or monthly categories) and the direct interview is essential for this.

The direct interview can adjust or omit questions which may be of a sensitive nature to the respondent. Without this flexibility there may be no response at all, but with a degree of understanding of a situation a considerable proportion of the questionnaire can be answered.

The major disadvantage of the direct interview is the cost of the exercise. Transportation, expenses, the wages of the interviewers and training costs are all higher than other methods. This is made worse if when specific, named members of a household are required because they may only be available in the evenings, thus adding to the collection costs.

The involvement of another human can introduce bias. The way questions are asked may even influence a response. Any major differences in socio-economic group, accent and appearance between interviewer and respondent could introduce subconscious bias. This is why if at all possible the questions should be asked exactly as printed on the questionnaire.

Increased concern about personal security makes obtaining access to someone's home increasingly difficult. Many people these days are extremely suspicious of strangers and will not answer the door under any circumstances. In such cases it is advisable to forewarn the respondents either by telephone or letter that an interviewer will be calling at a specific time. Another factor that makes personal interviewing difficult is that many people view any official visit to be connected with taxation demands and will thus be reluctant to even admit to living at a given address.

2. *Planned observation*

Some researchers use uncontrolled observations as a research tool but in the health sciences it is more common to control the observations from the outset. By living amongst the respondents, uncontrolled observations can provide fruitful material for future, more controlled measurement. Uncontrolled observation is very dependent on the personal skills of the observers and therefore lacks some of the scientific rigour required in experimental designs.

For controlled observation to be successful it is first necessary to provide a clear definition of the units to be observed and the information to be recorded.

The specific data for observation then has to be selected. The conditions for the observation need to be standardized. These will include the place, the time, the subjects etc. It is preferable to use electronic or mechanical devices and other methods of improving the accuracy of data collection such as video and turnstile entry counters.

Exercise 8.1

You require information on the level of patient interest in a health promotion video which is running on a continuous loop in a busy doctors waiting room. Describe the methodology you could employ to observe how patients view the video while it is being shown. You will need to record the degree of concentration, the *pro-rata* involvement, the effort made to view in relation to the position of the screen, etc.

3. *Recorders*

Video technology has provided great opportunities for planned observation because of low recurrent costs and the ability to replay in either slow or fast motion. Clinical psychologists commonly use special interview rooms with one way mirrors as an observational tool.

Electronic devices attached to televisions enables a central computer to record the time and channel watched. In health science research this could produce information on a specific advertising campaign such as HIV-Aids or solvent abuse, both of which have been featured recently. Although such devices are expensive to install, they have the advantage of being able to generate large amounts of very specific information and can show trends over time.

Electro-mechanical recorders are commonly used in traffic flow investigations and although their use in rarely *specific* to health science, applications in pollution control, occupational and environmental health are distinct possibilities.

Opto-electric sensors which record when a person has passed a given point would be of great value in determining movement of personnel in a hospital prior to redesigning a building. Clearly the errors produced by non humans such as trolleys, empty wheelchairs, etc would have to be taken into account when using such simple scoring techniques.

Computer technology allows more complicated recordings to be made. Surveys of health centre or hospital usage can be conducted by a single receptionist assigning each client into a pre-defined category. This can yield valuable information concerning waiting times, peak and off-peak periods, use of services (some people actually go into hospitals just to buy a cup of tea) and the numbers of people who are not receiving treatment but are accompanying patients.

Exercise 8.2

You are required to survey the use of a busy G.P. surgery using a personal computer. Produce a list of categories which may assist the practice to improve their services to patients. Assume that the operator (e.g. receptionist) only has time to operate two key strokes on the keyboard per individual. Remember as it is in a busy surgery the operator will not be able to ask many questions, so some such as age may need to be approximated. Having produced your list and assigned a key to each response, trial it with a partner on a real keyboard to see how intrusive the questions and computer responses may be. It is not necessary to write a program to store the data but you may on the basis of experience want to change some of the categories for it to operate more smoothly.

4. *Radio and television*

An appeal through radio or television is an excellent way to obtain subjects, especially for experiments of personal interest to the general public such as slimming. It is usually necessary to apply certain entry requirements to the subjects who volunteer but at least it is a quick way to obtain a large pool if available subjects. It is necessary to ensure that the appeal provides sufficient information to exclude unwanted categories otherwise the experimenter can expect to have to deal with an avalanche of enquiries. Ensure that if you give a telephone number adequate lines are available because often the response is overwhelming.

Radio and television can also be used to survey listeners' and viewers' responses to health issues but objectivity is bound to be reduced. Respondents' health knowledge can also be obtained through the medium of the radio and television, even delivered in the form of a quiz. It is essential if sampling is being adopted to ensure that the response is not biased by such things as the time of day of the broadcast and the capacity of the respondent to answer (e.g. availability of a telephone).

> *Exercise 8.3*
>
> Having delivered a health message concerning inoculation for measles on a local radio soap, you wish to establish how many listeners understood the issue. Write out an announcement for the radio station to attempt to elicit the information required. You are only permitted 30 seconds of air time repeated six times during the day. Take into account how the public should respond, how the responses will be logged and whether or not you need an incentive such as a prize draw.

5. *Telephone interviews*

Telephone interviews are increasingly popular as the proportion of the population owning a telephone increases. There is still a degree of bias because the poorer communities are less likely to be interviewed. However the saving on transportation and the advantages of conducting a personal interview without the problems of access are significant. An additional bias is that many companies sell products by "cold calling" customers and give the impression early in the call that it is a form of survey. It is thus essential to present your credentials early in the call to avoid that confusion.

The advantages of the telephone interview include speed, cost and success rate. A short interview can yield a very high number of responses per hour, and even allowing for engaged lines and dialling errors can be very productive. The cost, especially if local calls are used is far less than direct interviews, but of course the researcher cannot establish the same relationship with the respondent. The refusal rate, once a person has been contacted, is usually very low.

Another advantage of the telephone interview is that it can be timed to coincide with a particular event such as a 'no smoking day' or even with a T.V. programme. For example, a television documentary on healthy eating habits could be followed within half an hour by an evaluation on people's reactions to it.

The telephone interview is a very good way, by using postcodes, to control the geographical distribution of a sample. By the same token it is possible to cover the full spread of a large city without adding to the cost as they will all be local calls.

The major disadvantage is the representation, as fewer poorer people have telephones. It is also difficult to obtain detailed data as respondents become impatient if the call lasts too long. Attitudes and opinions are less likely to be given accurately over the telephone as a relationship has not been established between interviewer and respondent.

6. Postal questionnaire

This appears to be a simple method of obtaining detailed information at a cost effective rate. The respondent receives the questionnaire, is asked to complete it, and to return it. The response rate ranges dramatically with rates as higher as 57% and as low as 10% having been reported. A number of factors will determine the outcome including the length of the questionnaire, the importance attached to it and the use or otherwise of incentives.

It is possible to cover a wide geographical area at no extra cost. This especially applies if no direct interviews are used as a form of follow up.

Once the questionnaire has been produced there are no costs for staff training, travelling and wage costs.

The responses may be more honest if anonymity is assumed. Also a more considered response may be forthcoming because the respondent has time to complete the questionnaire and can check on facts (e.g. immunization records) if they are not known. The opportunity is also given for consultation with other people, especially family members, so it may not be a truly personal response.

The major concern of postal questionnaires is that the respondents will not be representative of the target group. This is primarily because unmotivated people will not respond, people move addresses or are away temporarily. It has been shown repeatedly that the highly opinionated and people who are well organized are the best respondents. It is essential, therefore, to have as an absolute minimum a number of follow-up letters. A postal questionnaire needs to have built into it a strategy to reduce the non response bias. Postal questionnaires can also suffer from misunderstandings of questions and accidental omissions (e.g. two pages turned over at once). The analysis must be capable of dealing with unanswered questions otherwise the whole questionnaire becomes redundant.

The length of a postal questionnaire is ideally short although for a major investigation such as a health survey this may not be possible. A maximum length of 11 pages is recommended but the presentation of the questions on each page will be equally important. It is almost impossible to judge the honesty and reliability of a postal questionnaire response.

The databases used to obtain the addresses of respondents are notoriously inaccurate. The electoral register in the UK was heavily influenced in the period 1990–92 by lack of registrants concerned about paying the community charge. A recent survey using a family health services authority database suggested that at least 50% of the addresses were incorrect.

After the initial flush of respondents from a postal questionnaire, the remainder will often take a long period to be returned. This means that plenty of time needs to be allowed and increasing effort has to be made to obtain responses from the last one third of the intended target group.

The style of a postal questionnaire will be slightly more limited than with a direct interview because it has to be capable of self-completion. This means that certain forms of questions used in oral methods such as case histories, extended conversations and unstructured interviews are inappropriate, but most other questioning styles are possible.

Open-ended questions can be used but are very difficult to code for computer analysis. Recall, recognition and coincidental questions are rarely appropriate because the timing of the survey cannot be guaranteed to coincide with the event being evaluated.

Dichotomous questions such as:

"Do you smoke?" Yes [ ] No [ ]

need sometimes to be supplemented by a "Don't know" option. This type of question is clearly the simplest one to analyze statistically but may not provide the depth of information always needed.

A check-list question such as:

Which of the following did you undertake last week?

Golf [ ]
Jogging [ ]
Badminton [ ]
Swimming [ ]
Cycling [ ]

is a common approach. However it is essential to ensure that adequate completion instructions are provided such as:

"Tick one box only".

Items can also be ranked such as:

"*Indicate how important to you are the following attributes of a physiotherapist*"?

Place (1) beside the most important, (2) next in importance etc.

[ ]	Knowledge of anatomy
[ ]	Pleasant manner
[ ]	Smart appearance
[ ]	Experience of equipment
[ ]	Technical skill

One disadvantage of this type of question is that no assumption can be made about the size of interval between the items in the ranks. Item 3 above (smart appearance) may be of no consequence and although it will get the lowest ranking is still only one rank behind another feature which may be considered of great worth by many respondents.

Multiple choice questions are often in the form of point rating scales and less commonly as graphic scales. A three point rating scale on cholesterol screening may ask:

"*How important do you consider it is to offer cholesterol testing to all middle aged people?*"

Fairly important [ ] Not important [ ] Very important [ ]

It is possible to design the responses so that a numerical response replaces the words or phrases so the terms used in a five-point rating scale such as *strongly approve, approve, undecided, disapprove and strongly disapprove* could be replaced with +2, +1, 0, -1 and -2.

The graphic rating scale allows the respondent to make a mark on a continuum to demonstrate strength of opinion, e.g.

Definitely approve	*Undecided*	*Definitely disapprove*
+10	0	–10

This method does make analysis more difficult but can provide a more sensitive scale for determining strength of opinion.

As a general rule questions should be worded by using simple words which will be familiar to the respondent. This is especially important in multi-ethnic samples when it may even be necessary to translate the whole questionnaire into different languages. The questions should be as short as possible yet obtain the exact information needed. Each one should only cover one point and be unambiguous. Leading questions should be avoided and prestigious names should only be included sparingly. For example “Do you approve of alternative medicine?” is a better option than “Do you approve of alternative medicine as recommended by Prince Charles?”. Certain words have emotional connotations and should be avoided. Political parties come into this category as do trade unions. One also has to be cautious about using questions that may be seen to reflect on the attitude of the respondent. Most people like to think that they are intelligent, witty, pleasant, good drivers, etc and will respond in a manner *expected* of them. One common fault is not allowing for all possible responses. This is why the *“Don’t know”* and *“Other (please specify)”* responses are so important. When using multiple choice questions it is essential to make the alternatives realistic. If not, a five - choice question effectively becomes a four -choice question and then comparisons with others becomes more difficult. All questions should be phrased so that the respondent has to use the minimum amount of writing. Ticks, crosses or numbers are the simplest and best form of response.

Questions should be arranged in logical groups such as demography, personal habits, health issues, nutritional knowledge, etc and not move around from one aspect to another. This is because people orientate to a particular aspect and don’t want to have to change their thoughts too often.

It is essential to start with simple questions so that the respondent is placed in a positive frame of mind. You do not want an antagonistic attitude created because the questions were too difficult. Questions of any embarrassing nature (salary, sexual preference, health habits) should be placed in the middle of the questionnaire so that a degree of rapport is established first.

Each question should be numbered consecutively so that coding and cross reference is made easy. Always allow enough space for entries, remembering that people write larger than typescript. If answers are linked to boxes for responses use dotted lines between them to ensure that no confusion can occur.

Give plenty of space between questions or divide by solid lines, bold face, etc. Emphasise key words with a different typeface such as italics. Items should be arranged in clear columns or rows to ensure that any not filled in can be spotted immediately.

7. Survey panels

This involves making more than one contact with the groups being surveyed. This longitudinal dimension provides information which cannot be obtained cross-sectionally. It will indicate more accurately the true trend in a phenomenon and not have the bias of different groups with the selection methods compounding the errors. It is especially useful if a specific strategy has been introduced which will effect the measure being considered. Physical recreation habits of sports centre users, for example, could well have been influenced by changes in management policy caused by compulsory competitive tendering. Panels of respondents surveyed annually during these policy changes will provide a clearer insight into the outcomes than would other methods.

Data gathered over time from the same people can demonstrate the stability of such measures when there is no apparent change. Profiles of individuals can also show up causal relationships which were not apparent in a single survey and can provide corroborative evidence for any which were shown at the initial stages.

Regular contacts with panel members may establish a relationship which enables more useful data to be obtained compared with a single visit. It also gives the opportunity for co-operative panels to become part of further experimental procedures.

The main disadvantage of the survey panel procedure is that the panel members will reduce over time. Respondents die, become ill, move house and no longer wish to continue for a number of reasons. This can mean that a group that was originally representative is no longer. Maintaining interest can be aided by regular feedback to respondents and cash or prize incentives. Starting with a group size much larger than eventually required will help and careful choice (e.g. respondents who are less likely to move and are younger) will also keep numbers higher providing that process does not introduce bias.

Sampling Methods

It is rare to be able to measure a complete population, although selected information on a *specified population* (e.g. age of death from myocardial infarction in the Wirral) is possible. It is more common to examine a *sample* from a population. This will only provide information on the sample itself, but if the sample were truly representative of the population it is possible *to infer* the population characteristics. If the sample is not representative of the population it is said to be *biased* and it would not be possible to infer population characteristics. The best way to avoid bias is to apply some form of randomization and all the examples that follow include this element of randomness.

Simple random sampling

This requires a full list of the population under consideration which is not easy to obtain. The electoral register is a common population database for adults but with the introduction of the community charge a significant proportion of the population have failed to register. The Family Health Service Authority (FHSA) database is a record of all people registered with general practitioners and is a reasonable representation of the population. It is also subject to inaccuracies associated with people leaving the area and not registering elsewhere or people failing to register in the first place.

It was estimated before the community charge was instituted that about 11% were not listed. However a much higher proportion of particular groups such as those recently moved (30%+), those in the younger age group (20% of those aged 25–29) and non-British citizens (49%) were not registered. Even if the electoral roll is used purely to supply addresses, undercoverage exists with the same sub-groups being poorly represented. Geographical differences also exist with 4% of the population being missed on average, but the figure rises to 6% in Wales and the South West and to 9% in inner London.

More specific populations such as patients entering a casualty department can be obtained directly from hospital records, but clearly a population comprising every patient from one hospital may not characterize other casualty departments. However the population is defined and obtained, it is commonly called the *sampling frame*. Once this is established, subjects are selected from the sampling frame at random. This usually involves the use of random number tables or generating the subjects randomly using computer software. The process continues until the required sample size is met and this will most often depend on the human and physical resources available to undertake the survey. The outcome should be a mix of subjects of different ages, fitness, health, shape, socio-economic status, etc. and should closely reflect the total population.

Systematic sampling

The difference between systematic and simple random sampling is that the subjects are selected from the population list in a *systematic* manner commonly at a set numerical interval. For example if a sample of 30 subjects were required to complete a student evaluation report on a course containing 150 students, every fifth student would be selected. The starting point for the selection of the first student would be obtained randomly by using random number tables.

Stratified sampling

Stratified sampling occurs when it is desirable to ensure that the sample has specific characteristics which represent the population as a whole. A common example would be gender where it is necessary to ensure that the sample has the same proportion of males and females. To obtain this, the sampling frame is divided into two homogeneous groups (e.g males in one group, females in the other) and then each group is randomly sampled. This will ensure an equal number of males and females which may not have occurred by simple random or stratified methods. It is possible that the sampling frame already has a particular characteristic that needs to be replicated in the sample. Gender in elderly people is, for example, heavily skewed towards females. It would be possible in a study of eyesight in the elderly to use stratified sampling to ensure that the correct sex ratio in the population was maintained in the sample.

Cluster sampling

Cluster sampling is used when there are administrative difficulties in testing a true random sample. For example, a study of lean body mass in Liverpool school children required a considerable amount of travelling between schools, organisation for parental approval, places to undertake the testing, etc. in each individual school. The budget and time available for the project was only sufficient to visit a sample of Liverpool schools and to measure the lean body mass of all children in those schools selected. This exemplifies the cluster sample approach.

Stage sampling

This extends the cluster sampling technique to further sampling stages. In the example given above, the head teacher of the school may decide that to test every child would be too disruptive but gives permission for selected children from certain classes to be tested. Thus having randomly selected a number of schools from the sampling frame the next *stage* is to randomly select certain classes from each school and then randomly select children from each class.

Volunteers

In human movement and health sciences it is common to recruit volunteers for surveys because it would normally be unethical to act otherwise. The consequence of this is that the sample will have some bias because subjects with certain characteristics will volunteer to participate whereas others will not. The most obvious features would be that volunteers must have the time to complete the survey, they must be capable of understanding the survey which usually means reading the languages in which it has been written. Certain personality types may prefer or decline to volunteer. In most cases little can be done to control this but it is essential that these aspects are kept to a minimum when a true random sample is required.

> *Exercise 8.4*
>
> Obtain a large population data set (e.g. electoral register, FHSA database, chamber of commerce business listing) and establish two sets of 100 subjects by (a) simple random sampling and (b) systematic sampling. Plot the geographical location of the subjects' home or businesses on a street map. Divide the map into regions and using the appropriate statistical test, establish if the method of sampling has made any difference to the geographical distribution.

Summary

1. Survey design is best validated by using a pilot study. One has to take into account the available finances, the time, the range required for the survey and the information content of the questions.

2. Information can be obtained by direct interview, by planned observation, by using recorders, radio and television, by telephone interview, by postal questionnaires or the use of survey panels.

3. The style of question is important and needs to be trialled appropriately.

4. Sampling procedures include simple random sampling, systematic sampling, stratified sampling and cluster sampling.

5. It is necessary to recognize the characteristics of volunteers.

PART III: *RESEARCH PRESENTATION*

Having concluded the research practice, the following three chapters and the appendices consider research presentation. Research which has been completed is of limited value unless presented to a wider audience who might gain from the researcher's findings. Chapter 9 is not concerned about the researcher's attempts to present data but to examine initially material which is already in print. This will often be the basis of current research and will represent research which has reached its final stage — availability in the public domain. Chapter 10 introduced the oral presentation and the research article, whereas Chapter 11 concentrates on the larger research report such as a dissertation. The two appendices provide rather specific information which will be of assistance for the research worker trying to publish for the first time.

CHAPTER 9

CRITICAL APPRAISAL OF RESEARCH

Key words : *meta-analysis; study purpose and nature; practicality; data record; bias; statistical content.*

Introduction

Critical comment on previous research is essential if scientific progress is to be achieved. It is easy to assume that if it is print, it must be correct. Most journals have a thorough review process; this is considered in Chapter 10 but the reader is best served if an article has been produced following a systematic critique.

Modern electronic retrieval systems provide such a breadth of information that a common tendency is to review the literature on abstracts alone. This is unwise and lacks scientific rigour. It is essential to obtain the main papers relevant to the study in their original and complete form. This in itself can lead to disappointment because an earlier or primary reference may then be needed to give specific details not available in the paper currently being studied. Frequently the assumptions and limitations of a technique are found only in the original with subsequent authors finding it more convenient to ignore such bothersome aspects. For example, much of the early body composition work, from which numerous subsequent equations have been derived, was based on a very restricted range of cadavers with a somewhat dubious representation of normality.

Having obtained the relevant article, it is essential to record its details and whereabouts efficiently. The most efficient method of accessing a database is to use keywords linked to specific fields such as authors' names or subjects. It will take time to establish such a database and many researchers are still content to use a card index system. The crucial decision relates to what keywords to assign to an article if a computerized method is to be adopted. The same applies to a card index system when the decision is either to use subject groupings or to settle for alphabetical storage by authors. The latter is acceptable if the researcher has the type of memory which can recall the author of an article. However as the number of references becomes larger this may prove difficult and subject-based indices may be desirable.

Some researchers find that with the judicious use of the highlighter pen an article can be reviewed and then stored. This process assumes that the correct information has been highlighted and the method of transmitting the critical information is efficient. Unless this happens the tendency will be for the article to be put on one side, re-read subsequently and the process repeated without significant transfer of information to where it is needed.

The main elements to examine in an article are:

1. Purpose of the study
2. Nature of the study
3. Procedure and research design
4. Technique of analyzing and recording data
5. Findings of the study
6. Interpretations and conclusions of the study

Each of these main elements will now be considered in more detail in the form of a number of checklists. It is not essential to *write* a full response to each question for every paper you read, but they should form the basis of, at the very least, a *mental* checklist. It would be a valuable exercise as an introductory researcher to take two articles and respond in writing to each question. You should by the end of the exercise have reached a far more critical opinion of the work.

Purpose Of The Study

1. Can you establish succinctly (i.e. in two sentences) the purpose of the study? An example would be "to establish the relationship between radiographs and surface measurements in scoliosis".

2. Is the topic related to a broader field of study? Are there any useful implications of the work?

3. What type of research is involved — e.g. basic, applied or action?

4. If the purpose of the study indicates an applied approach, does it suggest further applications or experimentation?

5. Does the study stay related to the purpose or do the researchers change to a different style of research?

6. Is too much proposed in the study so that the researchers cannot achieve their objectives?

7. Are vital terms defined adequately.

Nature Of The Study

1. Is the sample adequate for the purposes of the study. A small sample for a rare disease or condition may represent a large proportion of the available population?

2. How was the sample formed (see Chapter 8)? Were the subjects volunteers, hospital patients or formed in a totally random manner

3. Is the sample relevant to the total field of enquiry? Can the results be applied to a general population?

4. Is the sample or population involved described with precision?

Exercise 9.1

Spend five minutes writing a description of the people within your room. Start with the words "The subjects were...".
You may invent information about them as you will not have the time to take measurements or ask many questions. When the description has been written, exchange your attempt with a partner and see if a more precise and informative account can be constructed from the two individual attempts. A typical example is shown at the end of this chapter.

Procedure and Research Design

1. Were controls used and if so what type of control? In an experiment to establish the efficiency of a new drug, the outcome would normally be compared with a placebo as the control. However in certain designs it is inappropriate to withhold treatment and it may be necessary to compare treatments on the same subjects by giving two different types sequentially. Thus these subjects become their own controls. In critiquing a paper it is useful to examine how rigidly the controls are applied. Was careful matching undertaken for such variables as age, height and weight or was age the only form of matching applied?

2. How was the research constructed? What equipment was used? Was the research team suitably trained and qualified? What variables were considered? Were there any conflicting variables (e.g. diurnal variation, stage of the menstrual cycle, recency of previous meal) that were not taken into account?

3. Has the problem been adequately delimited? Were the constraints of the research fully recognized. Was the relevant previous research consulted with respect to the procedure and research design. This is especially relevant in surveys using questionnaires where there is a great temptation to start afresh. The limitation of this is that many questions provide similar information but because they are not asked in precisely the same manner, comparison cannot be made.

4. Is the overall research practical in its approach? Some research work may have been purely opportunist — e.g. a piece of equipment was temporarily on loan, a group of athletes was available for a single training weekend. Others may be impractical simply on financial grounds. This does not necessarily devalue the research but such aspects need recognition by future researchers.

5. Could the research design be re-created by others? This is of paramount importance. All accounts of research should be in sufficient detail for another researcher to be able to repeat the work exactly. This applies to such detail as the model number and manufacturer of essential equipment.

Exercise 9.2

Examine a paper from your own area of interest and see if sufficient detail is provided by the authors for the experiment to be replicated. The detail provided should be in relation to need. For example when a subject is required to watch a video-tape, the model number of the video-player may not be too crucial. However the size of the screen and the distance of the subject from that screen could make a great difference to the information content. Similarly "the measurement of body fat using an electrical impedance device (RJL Ltd, Gaithersburg)..." is insufficient because the manufacturer makes more than one model.

6. Were all instrumentation requirements considered? This usually applies to calibration procedures but may include following the manufacturer's recommendations. This is especially important when the state of the subject will influence the experimental results. In electrical measures of body composition, for example, the previous ingestion of food, drink and alcohol, the recency of exercise and voiding of urine may all influence the results.

7. Were the reasons for using specific procedures and equipment made clear? Were there, in your estimation, other methods which may have produced the same data, perhaps in a simpler fashion?

8. Were all pilot studies cited and well explained? Were they relevant to the present research design?

Techniques Of Analyzing And Recording Data

1. Were the data systematically recorded and well documented?

2. Was the presentation of the data (tables, figures) comprehensive yet easily understood? A good judge of tables and figures is whether they could 'stand alone' without cross reference to the text. Does the presentation of the data convey the information most effectively?

3. Was any data included that was not really essential with respect to the overall results and discussion? This is not uncommon and devalues the merit of a paper.

Findings, Interpretations And Conclusions Of The Study

1. Were the results interpreted in an unbiased fashion or were the prejudices of the authors apparent?
2. Were the findings well presented in a logical manner?
3. Were the summary and conclusions concisely and precisely stated?
4. Were the conclusions justified by the data gathered?
5. Did the author make a concluding statement in which the hypothesis of the study was accepted or rejected?
6. Did you consider that the authors were unprepared to commit themselves to any concrete conclusion?
7. Did the authors extrapolate their results to a larger population?
8. Did the study report any new questions that arose and make recommendation for further investigation.
9. Overall what were your views of the study? Were the findings too general, lacking specificity, or did you accept that this would be a necessary outcome of the research design?
10. What would you have done differently to produce more useful results?

Self Criticism

The above sections have been produced, as stated in the introduction, to assist in criticising existing research. However precisely the same questions must be asked of your own work. This applies while it is being undertaken, as the primary report is being written, and especially if you plan to submit the work for publication. The adage that if you point a finger at someone else you point three at yourself is never truer than in undertaking research. Use your critique of other workers to become a method of improving the scientific quality of your own research.

Biased Information

Although some information may be presented in a technically correct manner, the reader has to be aware of the possibility of bias. This is most likely to occur if work has been sponsored by a company with a vested interest. Few research workers will allow their judgment or their writing to be influenced by the funder of their research. However the information may be presented in a manner which looks perfectly respectable but fails to provide a true balance of opinion.

A considerable amount of health education material is now sponsored by the food industry and is readily accepted by schools short of teaching resources. The National Dairy Council produces nutritional information that advises pupils to have several helpings of milk and milk products daily. One has to assess whether this promotion, apparently based on sound evidence is acceptable. The Butter Council will argue that their education material is written by teachers and trialled in schools to ensure acceptability. This is no defence because the information on which the material is based may still be used selectively.

It is also very difficult to separate unbiased fact from good promotion. Dietary fibre may be promoted by a cereal manufacturer and polyunsaturates by a margarine company. They may both have a place in a healthy diet but the emphasis of each is where bias may appear.

Bias does not only exist where a sponsor or funding authority is involved. A private researcher may use the literature selectively to support the stated hypotheses. One way to avoid this is to undertake a *meta-analysis* of the research topic. This requires a thorough review of the literature using a computer-based system. The original references are obtained and the raw data, or if not available the grouped data, are combined and reanalyzed to obtain an unbiased view of the topic.

Statistical Content

A more rigorous critique of a paper involves checking specific areas such as the statistical content. Gardner, Machin and Campbell published two checklists in the *British Medical Journal* (1986, 292, 810-812) and part of these are reproduced below with permission from the authors.

Checklist for statistical review of general papers

Design Features

1.	Was the objective of the study sufficiently described?	Yes	Unclear	No
2.	Was an appropriate study design used to achieve the objective?	Yes	Unclear	No
3.	Was there a satisfactory statement given of the source of the subjects?	Yes	Unclear	No
4.	Was there a power based assessment of adequacy of sample size?	Yes	Unclear	No

Conduct of Study

5.	Was a satisfactory response rate achieved?	Yes	Unclear	No

Analysis and Presentation

6.	Was there a statement adequately describing or referencing all statistical procedures?	Yes	Unclear	No
7.	Were the statistical analyses used appropriate?	Yes	Unclear	No
8.	Was the presentation of statistical material satisfactory?	Yes	Unclear	No
9.	Were confidence intervals given for the main results?	Yes	Unclear	No
10.	Was the conclusion drawn from the statistical analysis justified?	Yes	Unclear	No

Check list for statistical review of papers on clinical trials

Design Features

1.	Was the objective of the trial sufficiently described?	Yes	Unclear	No
2.	Was there a satisfactory statement given of diagnostic criteria for entry to the trial?	Yes	Unclear	No
3.	Was there a satisfactory statement given of the source of the subjects?	Yes	Unclear	No
4.	Were concurrent controls used (as opposed to historical controls)?	Yes	Unclear	No
5.	Were the treatments well defined?	Yes	Unclear	No
6.	Was random allocation to treatment used?	Yes	Unclear	No
7.	Was the method of randomisation described?	Yes	Unclear	No
8.	Was there an acceptable delay from allocation to commencement of treatment?	Yes	Unclear	No
9.	Was the potential degree of blindness used?	Yes	Unclear	No
10.	Was there a satisfactory statement of criteria for outcome measures?	Yes	Unclear	No
11.	Were the outcome measures appropriate?	Yes	Unclear	No
12.	Was there a power based assessment of adequacy of of sample size?	Yes	Unclear	No
13.	Was the duration of post-treatment follow up stated?	Yes	Unclear	No

Commencement of Trial

14.	Were the treatment and control groups comparable in relevant measures?	Yes	Unclear	No
15.	Were a high proportion of the subjects followed up?	Yes	Unclear	No
16.	Did a high proportion of subjects complete treatment?	Yes	Unclear	No
17.	Were the drop outs described by treatment/ control groups?	Yes	Unclear	No
18.	Were side effects of treatment reported?	Yes	Unclear	No

Analysis and Presentation

19.	Was there a statement adequately describing or referencing all statistical procedures used?	Yes		No
20.	Were the statistical analyses used appropriate?	Yes	Unclear	No
21.	Were prognostic factors adequately considered?	Yes	Unclear	No
22.	Was the presentation of statistical material satisfactory?	Yes		No
23.	Were confidence intervals given for the main results?	Yes		No
24.	Was the conclusion drawn from the statistical analysis justified?	Yes	Unclear	No

These checklists have been designed to assess the statistical content of papers submitted to the *British Medical Journal*. It is unlikely that every paper read will be subject to such critical analysis by you after it has been published because it is reasonable to assume that the referees have considered most of these issues. However a mental checking of the statistical content of the papers read would be an advantage and the above guidelines do give an excellent evaluation. For those planning to submit material for publication you would be well advised to compare your statistical account with the checklists.

Typical Response to Exercise 9.1

The subjects were healthy physiotherapy students (15 M, 17 F) of mean age 20.3 (± 2.7) and mean heights; weights and IQs of 170.3 (± 5.6) mm, 70.2 (± 3.4) kg and 132 (± 27) respectively.

Summary

1. It is important to anticipate initial appraisal of one's own research and to be able to appraise others to make best use of it.
2. Critical analysis is achieved by asking a series of questions of every research report including the purpose of the study, the nature of the work, the procedure and research design, the techniques of analyzing and recording the data, the findings, the interpretation and the conclusions of the study.
3. It is important to recognize bias in a report and why this may be present.
4. Statistical content of a report involves design features, the conduct of the study, the design of the experiment, the details of the start of the trials, the analysis and presentation. Detailed checklists can help to establish whether or not your report or the one you are reviewing is of the required statistical standard.

CHAPTER 10

THE RESEARCH PRESENTATION

Key words : *preparation; visual aids; axes; delivery; instructions to authors.*

Introduction

All the hard work that goes into a well-constructed research project is of limited value unless it can be disseminated effectively. This takes a number of methods ranging from discussion with colleagues, informal seminars, formal oral presentations and submission for peer-reviewed publication. The importance of effective dissemination cannot be over stressed because a good piece of research can be wasted if not presented well. Presentation is crucial to business and commerce and should be no less so in the educational and academic community. It should not be the job of the listener or reader to unravel the important information from the presentation. This should be the task of the person delivering the message. Increasingly employers are demanding this of their employees. It should not be assumed that people are natural communicators but that certain procedures can be learnt and developed.

The key to any research presentation is to maintain the interest of the recipient and to be able to summarize the main points. Many academics consider that the use of simple ideas and illustrations is somehow demeaning and destroys their credibility. The situation is in fact just the reverse. Successful communicators can explain concepts and abstractions in 'down to earth' terms which are within the experience of the audience. A useful adage is "anything that can be said, can be said clearly".

The Oral Presentation

When asked to present research work orally, the style will reflect the audience and the relative importance of the occasion. Clearly a discussion over coffee with a group of fellow students or colleagues will require a different level of preparation and presentation than a formal presentation at a seminar or conference. In the former case the fundamental difference is that if things are unclear the opportunity will be provided for further discussion. This is rarely the case as the occasion becomes more structured. A conference presentation will set a time limit and opportunities for general debate will be limited although delegates may always approach the speaker later.

Students reading this chapter may consider that formal oral presentations are outside of their personal remit. This is not the case. Many institutions, for the reasons given above, require their students to present research work at least to their peers. Increasingly students are being encouraged to present their findings at appropriate conferences. The British Association of Sports Sciences has a tradition of welcoming student presentations and many learned societies do the same. Many students find the experience an ordeal but subsequently appreciate the benefits.

Although it is accepted that not everyone will have the opportunity to present in a formal setting, many of the principles apply to the informal gatherings. This book aims to raise standards and expectations so it is without apology that this chapter includes information and ideas which may appear at first to be the prerogative of the teacher not the taught.

Initial preparation

It is reasonable to assume that you are speaking because you have a greater knowledge of the topic than your audience. However it is sheer arrogance to assume that detailed preparation is not required. Well prepared notes will enhance the quality of your presentation and give you confidence, most especially if you are inexperienced.

The starting point is to be clear why you are talking. Is it to inform, to educate, to entertain or a combination of these? Sometimes it is legitimate to do little more than describe a technique. This would be when the development of the technique was the purpose of the research. However in most studies, it is the *results* of the research which should be emphasized. A very common fault in less experienced presenters is to spend too much time on the methodology to the detriment of the results. Assume your audience want results and be prepared to spend as much time as is necessary to transmit the results clearly.

The major constraint to any research presentation will be the *time* available to you. No chairman should tolerate a speaker going over time so you should establish well in advance how much time is to be given to your talk. Establish what proportion of the available time is for questions. It is common in scientific presentations for a 20 minute time allocation to be divided into 15 minutes for the presentation followed by 5 minutes for questions. The time will then condition how much you can say, and it is essential that you do not run over time. There is nothing more frustrating for an audience to hear a speaker say "I seem to have run over time so will have to stop here" when a summary or concluding statement has yet to be given. This reflects inadequate planning and rehearsal and does little for the credibility of the speaker. It is far preferable to finish well within your time allocation and leave more opportunity for questions, although the best option of all is to time your presentation to perfection.

Note what you wish to say on index cards. They have the advantage of being sturdier than paper and easier to alter the order. The structure for health and human movement science research will be similar to a paper but the emphasis will be different. Unlike a written paper when the reader can stop, go over a passage again and spend time comparing figures and tables, the oral presentation is continuous, sequential and one opportunity only is given to examine the data.

Write out your *main* headings on the index cards as in the following example:

1. Introduction
2. Purpose of the experiment
3. Subjects
4. Methods
5. Results
6. Discussion
7. Conclusions
8. Acknowledgements

Having done that, start to subdivide these main headings into subsidiary headings if appropriate. Does the introduction, for example, mean introducing you and the topic to the audience or is it setting the experiment in context rather like the introduction in a written paper. An additional advantage of sub-headings is that if you have insufficient time to include everything, index cards can be omitted without spoiling the overall presentation.

The revised listings may now have sub-headings which look like this:

1. Introduction
    - (i) Thanks for invitation
    - (ii) Title of presentation and co-workers
    - (iii) Interest in area of research

2. Purpose of the experiment
    (i) Main purpose
    (ii) Subsidiary purposes

3. Subjects

4. Methods
    (i) The criterion method
    (ii) The other methods

5. Results
    (i) Scatter diagram
    (ii) Correlation matrix
    (iii) Prediction equation

6. Discussion
    (i) Comparison with other studies
    (ii) Application to wider population

7. Conclusions
    (i) Relationship of findings to original hypotheses
    (ii) Specificity of results

8. Acknowledgements

Note that the subjects and the acknowledgements headings were not subdivided as they were complete sections.

These sub-headings then give the basis for adding the more detailed notes from which the presentation will be given. Some of the notes will be written but others may be in the form of illustrations. The results, for example, may take the form of three graphs, a correlation matrix derived from the graphs and a single regression equation relating the variables examined. Each of these would be on OHP acetate sheets or 35mm slides.

Although the use of index cards and notes are strongly advocated, there may be a case for preparing your presentation by writing it out in full. This will enable a concentration on the clarity of style and give you a better feel for the length of the presentation. Keep sentences short and personalize it by using the first person. Then check that every sentence is essential and if not remove it. Every 1,000 words is equivalent to about 10 minutes speaking time, but if diagrams are to be included this number decreases appreciably because adequate time must be given to figures to obtain the best from them. This fully written version is only a stage in the preparation and should not be used in the final presentation as scripts that are read come over far less satisfactorily than those based on notes. It is legitimate to read short sections, perhaps when it is necessary to quote exactly or a very difficult concept has to be stated without error. The full script can always be retained as a back up, just in case of 'drying up', but you should now return to developing your index cards as 'cue cards' for your presentation. The Physiological Society insist on the use of cues by having regulations which forbid an oral presentation being read.

Introduction

Most chairpersons will introduce the speakers and the topic but it is good practice to have an opening slide/acetate which gives the title and the researchers' names. To go straight into the purpose of the study would appear to be the logical next stage but this is assuming the audience are interested in the topic and if not are ready to concentrate on your area of research. The realism is that the audience may be settling down, trying to find the abstract in the proceedings or recovering from the dull presentation that has just finished. It is thus recommended to precede the statement of the purpose of the study with an *approach to the audience*. This device is really to orientate the audience to you as an individual. Jokes can be effective but because they are unexpected amongst scientific presentations often fall flat. An amusing response to the chairperson's introduction can help to concentrate the audience's attention. After a flattering introduction from the chair, for example, the speaker may say "I wish to say two prayers of forgiveness, one for the chairman for his exaggeration, and one for me for enjoying it so much". Alternatively a contentious statement related to the topic could make the audience pay attention e.g. "Some statisticians have shown no causal link between lung cancer and smoking". The contentious statement must be based on fact, but need not be a general consensus. Headlines from certain tabloid newspapers are often ideal e.g. "Mersey region waiting lists are the shortest in the country".

Once having gained the attention of the audience it is useful to set the context of the research to be described, preferably building on the broader knowledge of the audience. e.g. "You are all familiar with the government's consultation document on *The Health of the Nation.* I plan to concentrate on one issue — the lack of statistics describing the physical activity level of the UK population". The introduction should take about 10% of the available time.

Main part

The purpose of each experiment should be briefly explained within the overall context.

The methodology including the subjects and experimental design should be explained clearly and without great detail. This can be expanded during the questions. Any complex design needs a summary diagram, especially if different treatment conditions are being applied sequentially. A simple histogram with the x axis showing time can explain when blood was taken, when drugs were given, how long the pre-treatment period lasted etc.

The results, if quantitative, are usually best presented in the form of visual aids. Only the most receptive audience can retain numbers in their head when you move on to other aspects. If the results are on the screen in front of the audience, trends can be seen and the relationship of the variables can be appreciated.

The discussion section places the results in a broader context and must relate to the original hypotheses. Like other aspects of the oral presentation, the speaker needs to be briefer and clearer than in a written report.

The main part of the presentation should take approximately 80% of the time available.

Conclusion

This is an opportunity to bring the presentation to a close by summarizing the main points and emphasizing any part of the work which is needed. Do not introduce any new material at this stage. It is normal to acknowledge any special contribution made by others or from research funding at this stage. The conclusion should take about 10% of the time available.

Visual aids

The importance of good quality visual aids cannot be overstated. There is little point in presenting material which cannot be read easily. The most common fault is putting too much material on a slide or acetate. A table or graph that is acceptable in a written report may be totally inappropriate for an oral presentation. Limit each slide to a maximum of 6 lines of text or a table of six columns and three rows. The landscape shape is preferred to portrait. Each figure or table should have a clear heading. If using figures such as microscope slides or radiographs label them to direct the audience to the important information.

Before the talk

Having prepared your talk and having collated your slides or acetates the next stage is the rehearsal. This allows the timing to be checked. It re-assures you that the slides etc. have been prepared correctly (spelling mistakes do happen and are embarrassing in public), and more importantly allows criticism of the proposed presentation. Self-criticism is important but the research worker may be the last person to see imperfections. Ask fellow students, colleagues or partners to listen to a full rehearsal and comment on it. The writer has never known a rehearsal not to improve a presentation. If the speaker trips over words it may reflect too complex terminology. It will demonstrate the time lost through switching projectors on and off and help judge the required pace.

Concentrate especially on the figures, not forgetting that the speaker is familiar with the material and the audience is not. Spend time describing the *axes* of graphs because without the audience appreciating this the rest is meaningless. It is surprising how often a speaker will put up a graph and immediately say "you can see from this how x relates to y". It is far preferable to say "the horizontal axis refers to x going from a to b and the vertical axis refers to y going from c to d" before examining the data.

Once you are confident that your presentation is well-rehearsed it is useful to keep the slides in the carousel. This avoids slides being lost, crushed or re-arranged in transit.

Final preparation

If it is possible to do so in advance, the more information you can collect about the venue and the audience the better. How many people are expected in the audience, what previous knowledge do they have, how strict is the chair on timing, etc is useful background information.

More importantly "what is the room size?", "is the blackout adequate?", "where are the light switches?", "who receives your slides?", "how do you switch on the OHP" and "is there a pointer?" are all necessary questions.

If you are using visual aids, it is always worth having a final run through in the room you will be using. This is the only way you can get a final feel for your lecturing position relative to the screen.

Delivery

Having prepared thoroughly you should have the confidence to deliver your lecture in a pleasing manner. Detailed but misguided preparation can result in a speaker reading word for word from a script and wondering why the audience loses interest.

The rate of delivery is commonly too fast in inexperienced speakers. The force of the voice should be sufficient for the back row to hear it comfortably. The pitch should vary as appropriate with a monotone recognized as something to avoid at all costs.

Posture tends to be difficult to coach but can relax the speaker and audience if the speaker looks natural. It is a question of finding a compromise between being too stiff and excessively informal.

Lack of gestures looks unnatural but excessive movement can be disconcerting. Fluent movement to point to slides is desirable and special gestures to make a point has to be more expansive in a large lecture theatre to be effective.

Eye contact is essential to give the audience the feeling that the speaker is genuinely interested in the delivery and its impact. The speaker who finds this difficult should concentrate on one or two individuals and speak directly to them.

The Research Article

Writing up the work is an essential part of the research process. Research is not complete until it is published. Many students may not have this level of expectation but increasingly, especially as dissertations are prepared in a style more akin to a paper, the potential for publication exists. It is very sad to see many dissertations collect dust on library shelves when a limited amount of 'revision and reduction' could have made them suitable for publication.

Having established that an article is to be written the first stage is to make notes on what question has been asked. This can be expressed alternatively as what hypotheses have been suggested. This is followed by what conclusions have been reached. It is only when these two questions can be answered satisfactorily that it is possible to move to the subsequent stages.

Exercise 10.1

Select an article from a journal in your area of interest that does not have an abstract. Establish which questions are being asked in the article and what are the conclusions. This applied to other people's work is the process to be used in framing your own article. If the articles in your area of study all have abstracts then re-write the abstract, trying to make yours more informative. Aim for a length about two thirds of the original.

It is then necessary to select a suitable journal or magazine in which to publish. Magazines such as New Scientist have the advantage of a much wider audience and will accept shorter articles, but will not always accept uncommissioned material. Journals are the more common form of scientific dissemination. They are more prestigious because of the peer review process where all submissions are refereed by authorities in the area of study. The criteria to judge a journal may include the general quality and prestige, the size of the audience, the type of audience, the speed of publication, the rejection rate and in the case of radiological figures the quality of photographs. The most important criterion, however is the appropriateness of the journal to the intended content.

Exercise 10.2

Choose three journals from your chosen area of interest and by examining past issues find the publisher's statement on the policy of the journal with respect to content matter. To what extent do the journals vary or overlap and how would this assist you in making an informed choice? Next relate the stated policy to your assessment of the journal's articles. Do you find that the journal has strictly applied its own criteria or not?

The next stage is to write down the exact relationship between the findings from the research to be published and existing information. This could include where other people's work fell short of the present research, what specific advances have been made and what future developments may be possible. This starts to give an outline to the introduction and discussion sections of the paper and ensures that the proposed paper is justified in relation to existing publications.

A provisional title and a synopsis of the study can now be produced. This may seem strange for an article that has yet to be written but it is essential to focus the mind on the limitations of the study. The synopsis can take the form of the purpose or questions being asked, the observations or evidence and the deductions or conclusions. Do they all follow a logical sequence? This will set out the parameters for the article and provide the foundation for the subsequent more detailed writing.

From now on the writing will be concentrated on preparing for a given journal so this is the last chance to confirm that the scope of the journal is correct. Re-reading the publisher's statement will assist in this. Think in terms of the readership and try to consider their position. This will help in deciding whether material is too well known for the projected audience or lacking in the detail required.

The instructions to the authors should be read at this stage from the targeted journal. Some of this material will refer to details of copies to be submitted etc. but the order of the sections, the spelling, symbols, units of measurement, title pages, method of referencing, length of abstract, placement of figures and tables, formulas and equations are all information which is best learned prior to the detailed writing. If a page limit is not specified it is useful to gauge the length from previously published work in the selected journal.

The author should now be ready to establish the basic shape of the article. In the health and movement sciences this will normally be in sections of the introduction, methods, results and discussion. These divisions are not sacrosanct but have stood the test of time as being suitable for most scientific writing. Many journals will insist on that format, but if not it is reasonable to consider whether an alternative is justified. Any change from the conventional format should only be undertaken if the author is convinced that it will improve the article.

Once the sections have been agreed it is sensible to head separate sheets of paper with each section title. Brief notes can then be placed on each sheet with all the relevant information for every section. It is quite normal at this stage to mix fact, thoughts, ideas, comments and experimental detail. One can subsequently use a numbering system or linking arrows to create the correct sequence. However before this, it is essential to ensure that every item is strictly necessary. *Vice versa* has every item been included, and is every item in the right section? Some information could theoretically belong in both the introduction or discussion.

The tables and figures will have already been prepared in some form. Without this the author could not have determined that a publication was feasible. It is now necessary to produce them in a publishable form which requires a detailed title and legend so they can stand independent of the text. Research is all about results — the word should be written large on every laboratory door — and the efficient way to present them is by using tables and figures. Tables and figures provide an extended synopsis and will help decide whether the items noted earlier should be removed or increased. This is especially important when examining the conclusions. Can they all be supported from the facts available in the tables and figures?

The topic outline can now be produced for each of the major sections. This is when the fairly random jottings are put into correct order. In the case of the methods section it may be a chronological sequence of events. In the results section the most important may be placed first. It may be necessary to subdivide each section to make it clearer for the reader.

The next stage is considered by some to be unnecessary but can be especially valuable to the initiate writer. It involves constructing the sentence outline. This means taking each subject from the topic outline and making a specific statement on it. It is akin to writing a summary sentence which will be developed in full later. Judicious use of dots are appropriate at this state. For example information on the subjects could be written in sentence outline as "Subjects ... demography ...male/female differences ... numbers ... informed consent". Although a time-consuming operation, and not universally favoured, it can demonstrate any gaps in logic and indicate changes to be made before the first full draft is prepared.

The position has now been reached for a continuous attempt at the paper to be written. For a short article it is ideal to put aside sufficient time to produce the first draft in one session. This will generate a similar style and flow throughout the article. However it cannot be achieved if time is spent struggling for the precise wording on every occasion. It is better to omit words when this happens and fill in the gaps later. Advice differs in this aspect with some writers preferring to complete the more straightforward sections of the methods and results before tackling the others. As the introduction need only be short, it would seem no hardship to undertake that first, thus producing the first draft in the order of the final document.

The introduction does not need to be lengthy. This usually only demonstrates the writer's historical knowledge and that will be self-evident from the experiments themselves. An introduction need only include statements on:

(i) The general field of interest to orientate the reader to the topic

(ii) The specific findings of others which will be pertinent to the research work to follow, and

(iii) The questions which will be addressed.

If new techniques are to be used, the methods by which the questions will be answered can be mentioned. Fundamentally the introduction is scene setting and should tell the reader why this particular study was undertaken.

One of the biggest mistakes is to leave the referencing until the end. Although it is a nuisance to keep breaking off from writing the text to ensure references are written out completely, it is well worth it. Inevitably some detail will get mislaid and it is far better to document references clearly as the writing progresses.

The detail required for the methods and materials section is difficult to specify. It should be sufficient for the reader to be able to repeat the experiment exactly from the information provided. This will often depend on the needs of an experiment. As an example, a video recorder may be described differently in two different experiments. If the experiment was intended to measure the subjects' response to a videotape on smoking cessation it would be adequate to refer to a "VHS videorecorder" or a "Betamax videorecorder". This is because the videotape would operate on the one specified and as long as the subject watched the videotape the experimental protocol will be fulfilled. If, however, the style of observation became more critical such as an experiment in which specific eye movements were being noted in relationship to the screen, then a more detailed account would be necessary. In this scenario the statement may be "The subject sat 1.3m from a Panasonic "Profeel" with a 257cm screen which was the monitor for a Panasonic VHS videorecorder model 2880 ..."

Exercise 10.3

Obtain a dissertation from your department or library and condense the methods section into a form suitable for a journal.

The results section should be relatively straightforward as the figures and tables have already been prepared. Avoid repeating in the text what is already adequately explained in the tables and figures. Simply point out the main features and guide the reader to the important issues. There is disagreement as to whether conclusions should be mentioned in the results. Sometimes it is appropriate to make a statement concerning the implications of the results; at other times the results can be left without comment. What is worse is to re-state the results all over again in the discussion as a way of discussing them — a common error. Overall the results section should stand independently, with perhaps a hint of the author's intention prior to the discussion.

The detailed discussion will then follow which is the opportunity to broaden the perspective of the results and to re-examine the original hypotheses. As this is the 'meat' of the study, many authors find difficulty in keeping it short. However it must be recognized that the readership may not be as interested in the details as the author. Keep to the main argument. If the results turn out to be controversial this needs to be stated but a research paper is not the forum for personal vendettas. Be prepared to admit anomalies, even if a full explanation cannot be given. Bring out new possibilities for scientific examination which your results have indicated. It is reasonable to speculate within the discussion but it must be based on a solid foundation of observation. Although this must be a discussion of the results gathered it is also the opportunity to place the results in different contexts. The extent to which the sample may apply to a population can be explored. A study which showed, for example, that manipulative treatment for the back was not better but was quicker has broad ramifications for the finances of the NHS.

The first draft is now complete and it is time for the first revision. It is quite normal for revisions to be undertaken and arrogant to consider them unnecessary. The first draft has to be examined to see if any major alterations are necessary. Are there any flaws in the logic of the study? If the research has been well constructed then this would not be expected in the major hypothesis, but some of the minor hypotheses may no longer stand up to critical scrutiny. Take each sentence one by one and be absolutely sure that they are watertight in terms of the arguments being developed.

Next it is necessary to re-visit the literature. Check that any statement from every source is not only correctly quoted but is necessary and pertinent to the paper. Has every quotation been included out of sheer convenience for the author and is it quoted in the correct *original* context? This last point is important because a well-informed referee will know the original paper and will recognize inappropriate context.

Is the overall order of presentation, on second sight, the best? Would moving a paragraph make a more logical flow? Can tables or graphs be simplified or made clearer?

The next stage is a crucial revision process and involves a general improvement of the style, grammar and delivery of the text. Key features in the process include sentence construction, precision of every statement, clarity of terms and expression, directness and being concise.

Check the fog score (see Chapter 11) and reduce it to the lowest possible level by shortening sentence and long words. Avoid redundant terms like 'by some researchers' such as in the sentence 'It has been recognized *by some researchers* that coronary artery disease is related to poverty'. Remove all vernacular. Expressions which are acceptable in conversation are not always suitable for a written paper. Is jargon essential or can it be re-stated simpler? Particularly avoid a term which may be new parlance (e.g. waistcoat financing) but which may need explanation or may not be internationally recognized. Examine each word for precision of meaning and eliminate cliches.

Exercise 10.4

The verb "to vary" and its derivatives can cause confusion.

Discuss with a partner the precise meaning of the following pairs of statements and in so doing recognize how sloppy usage could confuse.

... plasma containing varying white cell concentration
... plasma containing various white cell concentration

... variety of improvements were shown
... various improvements were shown

... varied treatments were given
... different treatments were given

In scientific writing the abstract noun is used far too often when the verb would be better e.g. "Cholesterol determinations were undertaken by the dry chemistry procedure" should read "Cholesterol was determined by dry chemistry" or "Preferential release of lactic acid would appear to be common in ..." should read "Lactic acid is released preferentially in ..." One procedure well worth the effort is to reduce long lists of noun modifiers. "Exercise-induced asthma" is probably just acceptable. However if this were to become "high-energetic, exercise-induced asthma" or even worse "high-energetic, exercise-induced asthmatic subjects" one can soon see that the reader gets somewhat lost.

The final stages in producing the paper include re-reading the journal's *instructions to authors* (see Appendix 1) before the final typescript is produced. It is sensible to give this information to the typist, highlighting the areas which will be dealt with by the typist such as page size, font styles and paragraphing. It is your responsibility to provide the manuscript in as near a perfect form as possible so choice between roman or arabic numbering, underlining, upper and lower case can be presented to the typist. The last stage before the typist receives the manuscript is likely to be the final decision over a title and the abstract. Remember in reality many readers will not get beyond the abstract so it must convey sufficient detail of the study to help a reader decide whether the full paper is worth reading. This is especially the case with modern computer-based retrieval systems (or should that read ... with computer retrieval systems!) because often the abstract can be specified and printed. An abstract is sometimes confused with a summary and indeed some journals even use the terms interchangeably. An abstract should describe the whole paper and should be capable of being read without reference to the full text. The summary, on the other hand, reviews the salient points of the study and would be of limited value without reading the paper first.

Some journals will give specific details for producing an abstract but if not the following will be a good guide:

1. Title of paper
2. Authors (without titles). The lead author should be listed first unless alphabetical listing is specified (e.g. *Journal of Physiology*)
3. Institute or organization with full mailing address
4. A sentence statement of the paper's specific objectives
5. A statement of the method
6. A summary of the results which may include a table
7. A statement of the conclusions.

A limit of 300 words is common so unless otherwise stated keep within this number.

Exercise 10.4

Take a laboratory practical that has been fully written up using the conventional scientific design and produce a 300 word abstract using the plan shown above.

At the same time as the title and abstract are being produced any figures which need to be produced externally should be completed. Sometimes the quality of print is not sufficient for a journal and graphs have to be re-drawn. Indian ink drawings are sometimes necessary or radiographs have to be touched up to improve the clarity. It is often better to have this done by a professional and not assume that your efforts will be acceptable.

The final typescript is then produced and should be proofread. Proofreading is best done by the author in conjunction with a colleague or partner. This is because your own familiarity with the text may cause you to miss errors.

The typescript will be corrected and re-checked and then should be offered for critical review to different types of people. Someone who is intelligent but not at all familiar with the work will be able to spot stylistic limitations and the author's partner is ideal for this purpose. A person who is remote from the laboratory where the work was undertaken but is familiar with the work will be ideal to criticize the methodology, purposes and conceptual aspects. Finally, someone who was around when the work was being undertaken can make a contribution to the details of methodology. Such a person may notice some detail (environmental or procedural) which would have a bearing on the experiment but was not apparent to the researcher.

All this checking and double-checking may seem over cautious but it is far preferable than receiving a rejection from a journal which could have been prevented. It is not always necessary to accept the advice of colleagues but to have the comment at least gives the researcher the choice.

The final stage is to submit the requisite number of copies of the manuscript to the editor of the journal. Include a covering letter to ensure that the corresponding author is known and ensure that a request is included to acknowledge the safe receipt of the manuscript. This is usually undertaken automatically but without it you cannot tell if your precious cargo has reached its destination. Having received an acknowledgement the process of refereeing will begin and you must assume that this will take a minimum of six weeks. It is quite reasonable to make a polite enquiry if you do not hear from the editor after eight weeks — this may at least remind him or her to pursue a referee who has not responded.

Responding To The Editor

A straightforward acceptance without modification is rare but if it happens further correspondence is only necessary at the galley and page proof stage. It would be polite to indicate that you have received the letter of acceptance and look forward to seeing the paper in print.

A much more likely outcome is either a rejection or an invitation to re-submit the paper after modification.

A rejection by one editor or journal does not mean that the effort was worthless. A close examination of the referees' comments may reveal how restructuring will make it suitable for submission elsewhere. Alternatively it may require further experimental work before re-submission. Once again it may be best submitted to another journal after the additional work has been completed. A further alternative if you genuinely believe that the referee has misunderstood you or is incompetent, is to politely request the editor to reconsider. This has to be justified and is best attempted when two referees have given opposing reviews.

It is more common for a paper to be re-considered when revisions have been completed. This is not the same as an offer of publication subject to minor revisions. In the latter case the editor will often accept the revisions without showing it again to the referees. However major revisions will usually be submitted to the original or perhaps new referees.

When responding to specific referees' comments it is essential to cross reference each comment with your response. This can become very confusing if you are referring to the original manuscript (i.e. the one the referee has seen) and also to a new manuscript which is your re-submission. Respond to every point raised by the referee. If you cannot accept the criticism or it is impossible to undertake the recommendations then say so, but explain your reasons. If you accept the referees' criticism as being valid, make the corrections clearly indicating where they have been made. It is not the job of the editor to work out within a new manuscript where changes have been made. You should submit a covering letter which takes each comment in turn and explains your action. It must be recognized that the unknown and unpaid referee has given up his or her very valuable time to provide suggestions to improve the manuscript. Sometimes you may feel the suggestions are unnecessary, lack appreciation of the work and are even contrived. The fact remains that the editor trusts the referees and in the end if you want to get the work published you need to satisfy the editor. You must be assertive over issues that are important within the study and never prejudice your scientific principles. However it may be sensible to be conciliatory over small matters which are of less importance and thus establish a rapport between you and the publisher.

To help in your understanding of the way the referee might be thinking the following questions have been taken from the guidelines for referees from a well-known journal in the area of human movement and health sciences:

1. Does the paper sufficiently advance knowledge to merit publication?

2. Is the content of the paper within the scope of the journal?

3. Is the presentation sufficiently clear and precise?

4. Could the experiment(s) be repeated from the description and references given?

5. Are the illustrations necessary and adequate?
6. Are the aims clearly defined and followed?
7. Are the statistical analyses appropriate and clear?
8. Are the conclusions justified by the experimental evidence?
9. Are the references adequate?
10. Does the abstract accurately describe the work performed and the conclusions drawn?

Summary

Oral presentation

1. This requires initial preparation which includes knowing the time available and preparing appropriate notes.
2. The introduction must be designed to capture the audience's attention and 'set the scene' for what is to follow.
3. The main part of the presentation requires that the results are presented clearly.
4. The preparation of appropriate visual aids is crucial and the presentation of them requires practice.
5. Delivery is concerned with rate, posture, gestures and eye contact.

Research article

6. The editorial policy of the journal being considered and the instructions for authors must be read at an early stage.
7. The article is then built up as a series of sections with emphasis on the results. Subsequently the articles can be written or put together as a complete document.

8. References should be recorded in their entirety as the writing progresses and not left until last.

9. The methods section should be in sufficient detail that the experiment can be reported from the information provided.

10. The discussion interprets the results and introduces broader issues.

11. Attention should be paid to the use of the English language and sentence structure, especially the 'fog score'.

12. The proofread first draft should be offered for criticism to a colleague.

13. The checklist of 'guidelines for referees' provides an insight into the procedures adopted by referees of articles sent for publications.

CHAPTER 11

THE RESEARCH REPORT

Key words : *critical path analysis; supervisions; fog index; style; figure headings; student responsibilities.*

Introduction

Producing a full research report requires many of the same skills, information and approaches of a short paper. Indeed a number of institutions are encouraging students to present their research report not in the conventional formal of a dissertation but much more in keeping with a published paper. For the purposes of this chapter, however, the productionof a full length dissertation will be considered. The term *dissertation* will be used, but the same principles will apply to a special study, an extended study, a special report, a thesis or whatever term the institution favours.

Writing your dissertation is an essential part of the educational process. The discipline of putting pen to paper helps to focus the mind on the important aspects of the work. Often by writing things down, further thoughts occur and appropriate conclusions are formulated. Skills are developed along the way — those of critical reading, selection of appropriate material, assessment of the worth of results and the choice of the correct terminology. These and others will transfer to future careers.

Although all students will have a variety of forms of written assignment, the dissertation is likely to be the major, individual piece of work to be undertaken. For many, this will be the largest written report you will ever undertake and it therefore needs special guidance planning and preparation.

In addition to regular tutorials with your supervisor, it will be beneficial to talk to others who have undertaken a similar level of report or at the very least to examine previous dissertations.

Dissertation Requirements

Most academic reports have certain formal requirements such as the extent to which support can be expected, the degree of individual research and the amount of originality that is expected. Some studies can be 'desk studies' which are reviews of existing information, others are 'empirical studies' based on experimental approaches and yet others will combine the two extremes. All will have the characteristic of being systematic and require the results to be relevant to a broader body of knowledge than the specific topic chosen.

Some institutions specify a length, a format and a uniform style of presentation. These need to be known well in advance so time is not wasted on inappropriate preparation. Unless recent changes have occurred, the simplest way to establish this information is by reference to previous studies. Do not make the error of emulating another dissertation too closely as the model may not be a good one. This especially applies to the length of the report as an excessively lengthy dissertation will be criticized heavily. It is often more difficult to omit material which has taken time to collect but is sometimes necessary to avoid the criticism of padding.

Planning Ahead

The most efficient writing is based on systematic notes. Organise every unit of your project, whether it be the literature review or the experimental work, such that a clear, concise record is kept of what is undertaken. Do not rely on your memory. At the end of a hard testing session it is a great temptation to leave everything until the next day when you expect to be more alert. It is far better to spend some time immediately noting the issues that arose and checking that the results are stored carefully. An overnight cleaner may not be as discriminating as you and may destroy what appears to be scrap paper which in fact was a full day's data.

Nothing is more time consuming when you come to write up your reference list than incomplete references. Ensure that the full reference has been noted including the start and finish numbers of the page.

Some things, although undesirable, can be repeated, but experimental results cannot without a great deal of effort. Even then the laboratory conditions, the state of the subject and other environmental factors are unlikely to be identical. This means that extra security is required for raw data. A hard-backed book is far preferable as the first method of recording information than a loose leaf system which can easily come apart. It is always worth making a backup copy in case of loss or theft.

As data are being collected it is worth analyzing and interpreting it at the same time. This may help you recognize flaws in the methodology and plan better experiments to follow. The last thing you want is to reach the time you have allocated to write up your report and to find drawers full of raw data.

There is also a lot to be said for writing up parts of your report as you proceed. The methodology for your experiment for example, is much better undertaken while in the laboratory. All the equipment is present so you can record the make and model number, photographs can be taken and the detailed organisation etc. can be noted first hand.

In many laboratory or clinically based projects there are unavoidable delays with patients arriving late, equipment being repaired and subjects changing. On each occasion it will pay handsome dividends to develop the discipline to use that time to write up the study.

Planning The Whole Study

Although this chapter is mainly concerned with reporting the work, it is worth reviewing the many stages involved in the whole research project as writing up is only part of the whole process.

Many stages in the research process are contingent upon previous stages and inevitably a chain of contingencies is developed which ends in the final submission of the report. Not only is it important to recognize the links in this chain but how best to organize the individual parts in the most efficient manner.

The chains of contingencies can be treated in three ways:

1. To treat all activities as a continuous chain, tackling one task only after the preceding task has been completed. This results in a very long completion time.

2. To organize activities in parallel, semi-independent sequences where possible, avoiding the natural delays inherent in the simple chain. However any haphazard planning does not make full use of opportunities. Secondly it can result in not working at sufficient pressure early and then having insufficient time as the submission approaches.

3. To break down the total task into its logical sub-tasks and to arrange these into some optimal pattern. Such a pattern will need to cover all contingencies but can also achieve a better distribution of effort.

The method to achieve this optimal pattern is to prepare a *critical path analysis.*

Critical path analysis

The aim is to establish the sequence of contingent activities that cannot be shortened. This is the *critical path* that determines the minimum time from the start to the finish of the project. As there will be a pre-determined time limit, the critical path is established and then a series of parallel activities are fitted in to achieve the most desirable of the possible distributions of effort.

The model to be used to illustrate the process has the following characteristics:

1. Some kind of test material or apparatus is used
2. Data are collected using the above
3. The data are marked or classified
4. Statistics are computed on the processed data
5. Results are based on the statistics
6. Conclusions are based on the results.

The following rules are part of the model and will be followed:

1. No process may commence before its logical antecedents have been completed
2. No process *must* necessarily commence immediately after its logical antecedents have been completed
3. The critical path times must correspond realistically with calculated times for the activities. This rule will ensure successful critical path analysis work

The best method to establish a realistic task time is to:

1. Calculate the shortest possible time (most optimistic)
2. Estimate the longest possible time (most pessimistic)
3. Take the mean of 1 and 2

4. Moderate this in terms of known or expected factors (own work speed, work load, experience of delays, time availability, etc.).

If the task times exceed the total critical path length, either the task demands must be modified, or a decision must be made to reduce the task time, although there is bound to be a minimum below which one cannot go. In an industrial context it would be possible to employ more labour, but in research applications it is rarely possible to call on additional short-term resources. Parallel activities (e.g. a study of the related literature in the following example) can be omitted without affecting the critical path.

A list of most of the key stages in the process is as follows:

1. Decide the problem
2. Prepare the proposal
3. Read the first literature
4. Formulate the hypotheses
5. Design the experiment
6. Design the sample
7. Arrange for the subjects
8. Order the literature
9. Read the literature on hand
10. Await the ordered literature
11. Order the test material
12. Await the test material
13. Arrange the facilities
14. Write the method
15. Write the first literature review
16. Write the introduction
17. Read the ordered literature
18. Collect the data (test etc.)
19. Mark or classify the data
20. Type the introduction and method
21. Check the introduction and method
22. Compute the statistics
23. Assemble the final literature review and bibliography
24. Prepare the appendices
25. Write the results
26. Prepare the tables
27. Write the discussion and conclusions
28. Type and check the typing
29. Prepare, type and check the contents
30. Assemble and submit

Exercise 11.1

From the above list of 30 stages select only those which form the critical path and make a list. Then produce a timescale by placing the start and finish dates next to your first stage and your last stage and allocating an appropriate time to each critical stage. Include in your timetable any weeks when very little work can be undertaken because of holiday periods, other assignments, etc. The result should appear like the figure on the next page.

ONLY TURN OVER WHEN EXERCISE 11.1 IS COMPLETE

CRITICAL	PATHDATES
1. Decide problem	Nov. 10th – Nov. 13th
2. Prepare outline	Nov. 14th – Nov 17th
4. Formulate hypotheses	Nov. 18th – Nov 19th
5. Design experiment	Nov. 20th – Nov. 30th
11. Order test material	Dec. 1st – Dec. 3rd
12. Await test material	Dec. 4th – Jan. 9th
CHRISTMAS BREAK	
18. Collect data	Jan. 10th – Feb. 28th
19. Mark and classify data	March 1st – March 7th
22. Compute statistics	March 8th – March 15th
25. Write results	March 16th – March 31st
27. Write discussion and conclusions	April 1st – April 9th
28. Type and check	April 10th – April 19th
30. Assemble and submit	April 20th

It is now necessary to put in all the other stages which will run in parallel with the critical path. A final figure can then be produced which shows all the simultaneous activities and appears as Figure 11.2

Figure 11.1: Critical path timetable

Days in Week 1	2	3	4
1. Decide problem			
2. Prepare outline			
4. Formulate hypotheses	3. Read first literature	8. Order literature	
5. Design experiment			6. Design sample
11. Order test equipment	15. Write first literature review	10. Await ordered literature	7. Arrange subjects
12. Await test material		9. Read literature on hand	
18. Collect data			
19. Mark and classify data		17. Read ordered literature	
22. Compute statistics		23. Assemble final literature review and bibliography	
25. Write results			26. Prepare tables
27. Write discussion and conclusions	29. Prepare contents		
28. Type and check typing			
30. Assemble and submit			

Days in Week 5	6	7
16. Write introduction		14. Write method
	13. Arrange facilities	
20. Type introduction		20. Type method
21. Check introduction	24. Prepare appendices	21. Check method

Figure 11.2: Critical path analysis

Figure 11.2 shows you that at certain periods of time in the process you can have up to five different activities happening at once. Although the horizontal axis suggests days in the week, it is recognized that some activities will take longer than a day and adjustments have to be made to the time periods of the vertical axis as well. For example the period to collect data in Figure 11.2 has only been allocated one week which may be insufficient. What the critical path diagram does show, however, is that unless the activities listed are *considered* and *acted upon* sufficiently early, others in the sequence cannot be undertaken or a last minute panic ensues. This is often the consequence of a poorly organized student when many of the stages which should have been completed early in the process are left until the end.

When To Write

It can be seen that writing can be started at a very early stage in the study and indeed the discipline of writing focuses the thoughts in a most productive manner. It also has the advantage of giving the writer a basis for revisions and provides the supervisor with the report in more acceptable quantities. The critical pathway has shown that certain stages cannot be written up until the contingent stage is complete, but the big mistake is assuming that all the writing should be done at the end. Experience has proved that this will result in a rushed report. The quality of the final report will be dependent on the typing, the figures (including photographs) and the binding. Remember those things out of your control such as the binding cannot be recovered by extra work on your behalf. Assume that the binder will take longer than is promised and plan accordingly. Do not underestimate the time it takes to write your dissertation. If nothing else, preparing stages of the work in the form of a draft will indicate how quick you are at writing.

Supervision

Your supervisor should be a partner in the research process giving guidance and encouragement. The onus is upon the researcher to organize tutorials, provide information and report progress. You will not be penalized for regular consultation - just the reverse! Students are not expected to operate entirely independently but to complete stages of the work without direct supervision.

In preparing for a tutorial it is essential to provide information to your supervisor in advance, otherwise time is wasted while the supervisor is reading your material or reviewing progress. It is best to plan for regular short tutorials than occasional lengthy ones. At the end of each tutorial, agree on an action plan for the next few weeks and make an appointment for the next one.

Writing

Prepare each section by noting ideas, examples, information, suggestions, criticisms and conclusions. These notes can then be revised and placed into a proper structure.

Anticipate a number of alterations so if you are writing freehand, use alternate lines. Only use one side of paper to allow 'cutting and pasting' to occur later.

Short cuts are reasonable at this stage so use abbreviations. Text references can be coded with numbers to save writing them out in full at this stage but ensure the full reference is placed in the draft bibliography immediately.

The use of the word processor will save hours of time on subsequent revisions but ensure you always have back up copies. Be certain that you will be able to obtain a final copy at the quality of print required by the institution.

Clear communication is essential to disseminate your research effectively and this is best achieved by keeping your sentences simple and free of jargon.

Complex sentences full of pompous scientific terminology will only confuse the reader. Scientific writing is not only complicated by unnecessary jargon but is often poorly structured. A common fault is for sentences to be too long and contain too many lengthy words. A measure of sentence complexity is the fog index. It is calculated by:

1. Counting the number of words in a page of a given text and dividing by the number of sentences (i.e. average words per sentence).

2. Adding the percentage of words of more than two syllables.

The fog index for all Charles Dickens' books was less than 11, but it is not difficult to find official reports with fog indices in excess of 50.

Exercise 11.2

Obtain an official document from your sphere of interest and calculate the fog index. Compare this value with some of your own writing and from a piece of literature which you have enjoyed reading. Is there any evidence that a lower fog index is related to more pleasant reading? If your fog index is high, re-write the passage with more sentences and fewer long words.

It is common in scientific texts to use the third person singular past tense. The passive, impersonal mood e.g. "It was established that ... (Baltzopoulos, 1991)" is often preferred to the active form, e.g. "Baltzopoulos, (1991) established that ..."

Ensure that you establish the appropriate level of certainty. Many inexperienced writers confuse fact with opinion and are too eager to pronounce something proven. Quantitative results requires the significance levels to be stated or if non-significant for this to be recognized.

Having written a first draft of any section of your dissertation be prepared to allow others to see it. They may notice glaring errors of logic even if they are not familiar with the content. Others can certainly help with clarifying the meaning and noting typographical errors. Be prepared to accept that your style of writing is imperfect and to criticize it objectively. Complete the following exercise and having done so re-examine some of your own writing to see if any of the faults are found in your work.

Exercise 11.3

Analyze the following passage which contains examples of bad use of English and suggest improvements. Produce your own version before making reference to this author's comments which follow the extract. The sentences are numbered for reference in the commentary that follows. The names are fictitious.

(1) Following the recent appraisal undertaken by our consultants, the management has accepted the need for implementing greater Hospital integration with the Health Authority. *(2)* In order for the Hospital to present a common image it must show a consistent level of performance across all operating units particularly in terms of patient care and administrative skills. *(3)* To obtain this the Board has accepted that central management must play a greater part in directing each department's activities, although it is recognized that the autonomy of each department must be retained. *(4)* It is also accepted that significant increases in clinical throughput can be achieved in the short term by improving the overall Hospital standard of accountability. *(5)* The administrative control system should take into account the need for simplicity thereby maximising real patient contact. *(6)* The role of individual management will be to evaluate their respective operation, constantly and critically. *(7)* From this review the most appropriate system will be selected and then adapted to incorporate the specific operational characteristics of the Authority's Hospitals. *(8)* As the system evolves, it will be corroborated back to the individual departments in order to ensure comparability with national requirements.

Comment

(*1*) 'appraisal' of what?
'management' of what? Or should it be 'Management' with a capital M?
'accepted the need' : surely not! Recognised, perhaps
'implementing' : either leave this word out or expand the phrase to 'implementing our consultants' recommendation for ...'
'greater Hospital integration': this is unclear. The individual hospitals could be integrated into the Health Authority or could be better integrated internally. However, integration means loss of identity. Perhaps 'co-operation' or even 'standardization of procedures' was intended.

(*2*) 'In order for .. to' is clumsy and not standard English.
'common image': the Hospital, being singular, can have only one image. The individual departments could present a common image, i.e. all have the name image.
'consistent level': the same applies – consistent with what? The levels (plural) of the individual operating units could be the same.
'performance' of what?
'in terms of': one does not perform in terms, one performs in the thing itself i.e. in administrative skills. One does not perform in a skill, one has or develops or acquires a skill.

The whole sentence would have been clearer if 'operating units' had been made the subject and the more usual order used of subject/verb/object/dependant clause.

(*3*) 'To obtain this': what? Consistency of level(s)?
'accepted': This time the meaning is 'agreed'?
'play a greater part in directing': i.e. 'direct more of'.
'although ...' The second part of the sentence contradicts the first. If some activities are directed by an outsider then some autonomy is lost. If this autonomy 'must be maintained' then Central Management must play no part in directing. Perhaps what the writer meant to say

was something like ‘while it is desirable that the autonomy of each department should be retained as far as possible, there are some functions which must be directed from the centre’.

(4) ‘accepted’: This time the meaning is ‘believed’.
‘improving the overall Hospital standard’: Why not try something like ‘a general improvement in ...’

(5) ‘need for simplicity ...’: This is a non-sequitur as well as being bad grammar. It should presumably read ‘need to maximise patient contact’ (Whether a simple system will do this or not is not implicit in the need. A sophisticated system might be more effective. It depends on what is meant.)
‘real patient contract’: What else is patient contact other than real? Fictitious? Imaginary?

(6) ‘The role of individual management?: presumably what was meant was ‘each manager’. As it stands it is nonsense.
‘evaluate’: review would make more sense: or substitute.
‘Performance’ for ‘operation’.
‘constant’: i.e. at regular intervals.
‘critical’: This would apply to ‘review’ or ‘examination’, not ‘evaluation’.

(7) ‘incorporate’: i.e. ‘take amount of’.
‘specific’: i.e. ‘particular’.

(8) ‘corraborated’: obviously the wrong word. The writer may have meant ‘seen to be justified’ or possibly ‘need to be modified’.
‘comparability’: This looks as if it might be a typing error for ‘compatibility’. Alternatively the writer may have meant ‘to comply with national legislation’.

Once the stage of the final draft has been achieved you must now undertake the last round of revisions. These will include ensuring that the grammar, the arguments, and the spelling are correct and that the references are properly cited. If you use a spelling check routine on a computer ensure that the thesaurus uses English spelling for institutes in the United Kingdom. When citing references or quoting use the original spelling. It is incorrect to convert the *Journal of Pediatric Exercise* to the *Journal of Paediatric Exercise*. Ensure that all references within the text are correctly cited in the reference list. Likewise check that no additional references are quoted. The only way to confirm this is to tick off each reference on the reference list when you read it in the text. Because you are "close" to your subject you may miss errors. Ask someone who is unfamiliar with the subject area to check for typographical errors and poor style. If it is fully comprehensible to a friend or spouse it will be a better report than one which cannot be fully understood by someone who knows you well. Do not expect your supervisor to do this for you because this is the point at which he or she will revert to becoming your examiner.

Having produced the final manuscript the report will have to be typed. Allow adequate time for this, especially if the complete manuscript is handed over to the typist. It is preferable to provide the material in sections so that it can be checked in stages. However it is essential to confirm that the same typist will be available to complete the work as changes in typeface may be unacceptable. Ask the typist to provide a specimen of the layout and ensure that it conforms to the requirements of the institution with respect to the width of the margin, line spacing, indentation, etc.

The most preferable option is to have the manuscript typed on a wordprocessor. This means that any changes will not effect subsequent pages and necessitate re-typing. Do ensure that back-up copies are made. The main disadvantage of the wordprocessor is the quality of the eventual product. Has your typist access to a laser printer or a letter quality daisy wheel printer? If not, will the institution accept a near letter quality printer or a dot matrix?

Ensure that the dip switch settings are appropriate to your requirements. It is no excuse to have all '£' signs entered as '$' simply because the printer is not configured correctly. Mathematical symbols, formulae and foreign characters will occasionally not be available and these will need to be added later by hand in indian ink or using letraset.

Figures can include photographs, line drawings, charts or graphs. Photocopies of photographs are not usually of sufficient quality and each copy of the report should contain an original print. Line drawings and graphs can usually be photocopied to the standard required. The figures should be numbered, should have a title and also a legend. The numbering is sequential and easier to follow if the first number refers to the chapter. For example Figure 3.2 would be the second figure in Chapter 3. The title is a brief heading and the legend briefly explains the figure. An example from elsewhere is shown in the box below.

Figure 29.1

Time spent playing sport per week by male and female respondents

The vertical scale gives the percentage of males and females who played sport for the number of hours indicated on the horizontal scale.

References are essential to permit the reader to follow up details that were not possible within the report. It also indicates how thoroughly the literature has been reviewed. It is essential that references are quoted formally. In most cases the text will include the first author and the year of publication. If the reference has two authors only they are both quoted e.g. Smith and Jones (1991), but where the reference has more than two authors it is common to quote the first author followed by *et al*. The *et al*., being latin is italicized but if the typist cannot offer that facility it is underlined. Although some journals prefer a numbering system e.g. "It is believed that ......[19].", this is not recommended for a dissertation as any reference changes could result in a major re-numbering which would be very laborious.

The reference list appears in the bibliography when the complete reference with every author will appear in alphabetical order.

Appendices can be used in dissertations to include material which is useful but would complicate the main body of the text unnecessarily. Details of experimental procedure, informed consent forms and questionnaires are examples of material best placed in an appendix.

Student And Supervisor Relationship

It is essential in the production of a dissertation that the relationship between the student and supervisor is recognised and properly established. There is nothing worse than unrealized expectations on either side.

The supervisor has certain responsibilities which may include:

(a) keeping the student informed about developments within the area of the research

(b) providing guidance about the standards expected, planning, special techniques and organizational aspects which may include attending courses or taught classes

(c) being accessible when the tutorials have been arranged

(d) requesting written submissions on specified dates and returning the work appropriately marked within a reasonable time

(e) providing practice for special aspects of dissertation such as *vivas*, oral presentations, etc

(g) keeping students informed of inadequacies

(h) checking that students with special needs e.g. foreign students with language difficulties or disabled students, are catered for satisfactorily

The students' responsibilities will include:

(a) preparing the research proposal in sufficient detail for the supervisor to be able to accept each stage of the work in advance

(b) ensuring that any deviation from the proposal is agreed with the supervisor

(c) arranging regular tutorials. It is often best to conclude a tutorial with a plan of action for the next period of time and for this to culminate in another tutorial. Supervisors get very committed and it is wise to have your tutorial in the supervisor's diary well in advance

(d) raising problems, however small, with your supervisor if they cannot be resolved personally

(e) providing written material in plenty of time for it to be read prior to a tutorial

(f) informing the head of department of a breakdown of the personal relationship between the student and supervisor which will be detrimental to the outcome of the research

(g) writing the dissertation. This may appear at face value to be obvious but it is surprising how expectations can differ. A supervisor will wish to do his/her best for a student but it must be the student's work, even if after advice it is not of the required standard. Most failures are a consequence of a student not maintaining regular contact or not taking the advice of the supervisor.

Summary

1. There is no substitute for planning ahead and a critical path analysis is one method.
2. Key stages in planning the dissertation have to be identified and put into a time scale.
3. It must be recognized that certain aspects will run in parallel with others and that time for malfunctions and subject unavailability will be necessary.
4. Supervision is the key to much of this work and planned tutorials will often make the difference between success and failure.
5. Ensure that you clarify with your supervisor the aspects (s)he expects of you and you of him/her.
6. Poor writing can ruin a dissertation so make every effort to write clearly and accurately.

APPENDIX 1

INSTRUCTIONS FOR AUTHORS

This is an example of notes for authors for a specific journal (*Sports Medicine*). It is important to recognize that other journals will have special requirements which must be followed.

Special Note Re Applied/Clinical Content Of Articles

All articles are to be based on data or findings in humans which have relevance to practical application for sports participants or prescription of exercise. Data from animal or *in vitro* investigations can be included only if they have direct support for the topic under discussion.

Manuscript Preparation

Articles will be published in English. Submit two copies of the complete manuscript, including text pages, references, tables, legends, footnotes and figures. Only typed copy, double-spaced on one side of preferably A4 (206mm × 294mm) typewriter paper, and with liberal margins is acceptable.

Subdivisions Of Articles

Manuscripts should be prepared and paginated in the following manner:

a) Title page
b) Summary
c) Text pages

d) Acknowledgements
e) List of references
f) Address for correspondence
g) Tables
h) Figures and legends
i) Footnotes

Title Page

There should be a separate title page with title, authors and institutions where the work was done, indicating city, and a condensed running title of not more than 50 letters including spaces.

The name and address of the author to whom reprint requests should be addressed should appear separately at the end of the references.

Summary

The third page should contain a summary. The summary should be about 5% of the length of the article and should highlight the salient points discussed.

References

In the text, reference to published work is cited by author (alphabetically) and year – *viz*. (Hart 1968, 1972; Lind *et al.* 1970; Mariner & Jamieson 1966)... (Tipping 1982b; Wilson & Payne 1984b,c,d).

The list of references must be arranged alphabetically by first author's name (and initials if more than one author of the same name) or by second or third etc authors if more than one author of the same name and initials. If the sequence of the authors' names and initials is identical, the references should be arranged chronologically by year of publication. Five authors per reference need only be given.

Sample references are listed below. *Note*: titles of journals are *not* to be abbreviated. Supply inclusive pagination for all articles.

Journal: Hart AH, Harman GN, and Layne MT. Metronidazole kinetics in dialysis patients. *Surgery* 93: 149–153, 1968.

Wilson SU, and Payne YB. Aspirin consumption in North Wales. *The Lancet*, in press, 1984c.

Book:	Hart AH. Pharmacokinetics and metabolism of the benzamides. In Platts *et al.* The benzamides: pharmacology and clinical aspects. 3rd ed., Vol. 36, Raven Press, New York, 1969.
Supplement:	Mariner E, and Jamieson Jr HF. Beta-blocking drugs and sleep: a controlled trial. *Clinical Pharmacology and Therapeutics* 25 (Suppl. 2): 628–632, 1966.
Symposium:	Tipping NGW. Disposition of nitroglycerine in rat plasma. 8th Congress of Pharmacologists, Tokyo, July 19–24, 1981. Abstract no. 223, p.514, 1982b.

Tables

Type double-spaced on a separate sheet, number with Roman numerals (I, II etc.) and provide a legend for each. Tables should be comprehensible without reference to the text. Data given in tables should in general not be duplicated in the text or figures. Any necessary descriptions should appear as numbered footnotes at the bottom of the table.

Illustrations

Illustrations are referred to in the text by Arabic numerals (1, 2 etc). Legends for illustrations should be typed on a separate sheet, numbered correspondingly and should make the illustration understandable independently of the text. The approximate position of each illustration should be marked in the text.

For line drawings, good-quality glossy prints or black ink drawings are requested. For half-tone illustrations, well contrasted photographic prints, trimmed at right angles are requested. Symbols, abbreviations and spelling should be consistent with the text. Figures should be professionally drawn and photographed, if possible.

The author's name, the figure number and top of the figure must be indicated (lightly) on the back of each print.

Lettering and symbols on figures should be clear and large enough (14 point *sans serif* type is preferable) to be easily readable after 50% size-reduction. When possible submissions of figures already reduced to confirm to the column or page-size requirements of the journal will facilitate publication. In already reduced form, column width should not exceed 6.3cm and full-page size should not exceed 14.1cm × 18.5cm.

Abbreviations and Symbols

Use SI symbols and recognized abbreviations for units of measurement. The first time an uncommon abbreviation appears, it should be preceded by the full name for which it stands.

APPENDIX 2

FORMAT AND STYLE FOR REPORTS AND PAPERS

Most institutions will have a recommended format for their dissertations but may not have provided the detailed guidance that follows. It will be necessary, therefore, to take account of local regulations but we still consider it useful to lay out a procedure that can be followed with confidence if doubt still exists. This will equally apply to papers as indicated in Chapter 10 when instructions for authors should provide some information on format and style. An excellent publication is the American Psychological Association text entitled *Publication Manual of the American Psychological Association*, 3rd Edition (APA, 1984), which provides great detail on format and style. This Appendix is designed as a compromise between the more detailed texts such as the APA manual and the two page handout which is common in educational institutions. Slight adjustments will be needed depending on whether you are writing an extended report such as a dissertation or a research paper. This book has been produced in the following format so you can see what it looks like if you are following these instructions.

Equipment

Typewriters

If possible, use an electric typewriter with a carbon ribbon. If there is a choice of typeface, the preferred one is Prestige Elite 12 pitch. If a manual machine has to be used, obtain a fresh, black ribbon for typing the first manuscript.

Spacing

Type the text of the paper with single line spacing, unless your paper contains many subscripts and superscripts; in that case, use one-and-a-half (1.5) line spacing. Set the left- and right-hand margin stops to a width of 12.7cm (5"). Set the tabulator so that it indents 5 spaces, approx. 1cm, from the left-hand margin.

Word Processors

Printer: If possible, use a word processor with a laser or daisy wheel printer. If there is a choice of typeface, the preferred one is Prestige Elite 12 pitch, black.

Paper: Use good quality A4 size paper. The typing area for the text is 12.7cm (5") wide by 20.3cm (8") deep. Try to fill the area, exceeding the width by only two or three characters if necessary. *DO NOT, UNDER ANY CIRCUMSTANCES, TYPE YOUR TEXT TO FULL A4 SIZE PAGES.*

Spacing: Use single spacing unless your text contains many subscripts and superscripts; in that case use one-and-a-half or double-line spacing. Set the left- and right-hand margin stops to a width of 12.7cm (5"). Set the tabulator so that it indents 5 spaces, approx. 1cm from the left-hand margin.

Text Format

Chapter Headings

On the first page leave 5.0cm space from the top.

Title: Type the chapter title all in capitals (upper case), indented five spaces. If the title is more than one line long, indent all lines of the title by the same amount.

Author's Name (if required): Leave three lines of space after the title,, then type the full name(s) of the author(s) in capitals, indented.

Author's Address (if required): Type the author's address in upper and lower case on the line immediately below the author's name. Run on the address to make the minimum number of lines, and indent each line.

Abstract: If a concise abstract is required, not more than 300 words, leave two lines of space after the author's address, indent, then type the works "Abstract" and underline. Leave three typewriter spaces, then type the abstract, each line indented.

Key Words: The abstract, if required, may be followed by a list of up to six key words or phrases that between them indicate the subject matter of the paper. These will be used for indexing and data retrieval purposes. Leave two lines of space below the abstract, then type "Key Words", indented as for the abstract, and underline. Leave three typewriter spaces, then type the key words or phrases, with a commas between each one and full stop at the end. Each line should be indented. Leave three lines of space below the list before beginning the text.

Text Headings

All headings should be set over to the left-hand margin. Type first level (sectional) headings all in capital letters; put two lines of extra space above the heading and one line of space below. Second level headings should be typed in lower case letters, but with the first letter of each main word in capital. For third level headings, only the first letter of the first word should be a capital. Second and third level headings should be underlined, with one line of extra space above but no extra space below for example:

FIRST LEVEL TEXT HEADINGS

Second Level Text Headings

Third level text headings

Headings may be set in bold or italic type if these are available.

Line Length

For typewritten copy, aim at finishing each line as close as possible to the pre-set right-hand margin. If a word processor is used, make sure that no line exceeds 12.7cm (5") in width.

Paragraphs

Indent the text at the beginning of each new paragraph not after a text heading. When the text is started fill out to the left-hand margin. Do not leave any space between paragraphs.

Spelling

American spelling is usual for many international journals but English spelling is necessary for UK based reports. Whichever system is used, it should be used consistently throughout. For American spelling, use *The American Heritage Dictionary.* For English spelling, use *The Concise Oxford Dictionary* or *The Oxford Dictionary for Writers and Editors*. Note, however, the following:

Use "ize" not "ise" spellings

While (not whilst)	among (not amongst)	Postgraduate
coorporate	focused	cross section
pretreated	fetus (not foetus)	occurring
acknowledgement	judgement	microorganism
out-patient	*in vivo* (no hyphen)	

Underlining/Italic Type

Use underlining, or italic type if available, to stress words or phrases, and for the titles of books, films, plays, works of art, poems, periodicals, and ships. See also the sections on Foreign Words, Mathematics and Biology.

Lists

When listing items or points set them out in the following style.

1. Text. . . . .
. . . .
2. . . . .
. . . .
(i) . . . .
. . . .
(ii). . . . .
. . . .
(iii) . . . .
. . . .

Note the exact position of the lines of the text. One line of extra space should be left above and below the list. If the list is run on in the text, the numbers or letters should be in parentheses – e.g. (1)...........................; (2)...........................; (3)...........................

Capitals

Use capitals for proper names, titles, geographical names, trade names, etc.:
"Sir Peter Edwards, Earl of Gayton always drinks Pepsi".
Use a capital for the particular and lower case for the general, e.g:
Chapter 1, but in later chapters; the Church, the State and the UK Government, but a small church, an African state, a new government.

Compass points and regions: The North, Midlands etc., but five miles north of London, south-west.

Headings: In headings where all main words have initial capitals, mostly second level headings, the following are the kinds of words that do not take an initial capital (unless they are the first word):
a, the, in, by with, between (i.e. all prepositions), its, their, his. But if an italic (underlined) phrase is used in a heading, both parts have initial caps, even if one is a preposition — e.g. *In Vitro, Ab Initio*. The exception to this is with Latin names for organisms — e.g. *Escherischia coli* — which do not take an initial capital for the second part.

Seasons: spring, summer, etc. No capitals.

Hyphens

Hyphens are most often used in compound adjectives, e.g. well-prepared lecture, up-to-date report. This is extremely important when confusion may be caused if there are no hyphens; compare "three-day old kittens" with "three day-old kittens". However, if the adjective is separate from the noun, it is not hyphenated, e.g. the lecture was well prepared, the report is up to date. Also, if one word is an adverb, there is no hyphen: "a quickly made decision".

Abbreviations and Contractions

Abbreviations not in common use should be spelled out in full the first time they occur in a typescript — e.g. Greenwich Mean Time (GMT).
Names (of countries, institutions, honours, etc.) and *acronyms* are mostly abbreviated without full stops and without spaces between the letters. Examples: USA, UK, PM (Prime Minister), NUJ, TUC, BBC, OBE, FRS, BA. Those that are pronounceable are often written with an initial capital and the rest lower case.
Examples: Aslef, Sogat, Fortran, Basic.
Initials are written with a full stop - H.G. Wells.

Other abbreviations take full points. Examples: e.g., i.e., Inc., a.m., p.m., Yorks., etc., et al., Prof.
Contractions however, are not written with a full point (i.e. if the last letter of the word is included in the abbreviation). Examples: Ltd, Mr, Dr, Mrs, Ms, St (Saint). Exceptions include scientific terms (see under Measurements and Units) and chemical elements (see section on Chemistry). See *The Oxford Dictionary for Writers and Editors* if you are not sure about any particular abbreviation.

Foreign Words

Those that have not been adopted into the English language are underlined or set in italics. Examples:

ab initio	*hors de combat*	*object d'art*
ad hoc	*in situ*	*par excellence*
ad nauseam	*in vitro*	*per se*
circa (abbrev.c.)	*in vivo*	*raison d'etre*
coup d'etat	*joie de vivre*	*sine qua non*
en masse	*modus operandi*	*tour de force*
fait accompli	*nom de plume*	*vide*

Anglicized worlds, however, are not underlined. Examples:

alias	ex-officio	postmortem
a priori	fiance(e)	pro rata
apropos	in camera	regime
avant-garde	milieu	status quo
bona fide	mores	verbatim
creche	nuance	versus
curriculum vitae	per annum	via
debut	per capita	vice versa

If in doubt whether a word should be italicized, consult *The Oxford Dictionary for Writers and Editors.*

Quotations

Quotations set inside the text should be in double quotes, with single quotes used only for quotes within quotes. Interpolations inside quotes (i.e. if the author adds something of his own to the quote) should be in square brackets.

Punctuation: If a quote has certain punctuation, this must be kept inside the quotation marks; other punctuation belongs outside.

Poetry: Poetry, sometimes used for epigrams, etc., is not usually set in quotation marks, but as a separate block. It has a single line space above and below the quote, and can be inset or centred. The poet's name is often set below the quote, ranged right.

Qualifications

S.L.Pillow, BA, PhD, MD (commas between each degree but no punctuation).

Illustrations

All figures must be mentioned in the text, as "Figure 1" in full, not "Fig. 1". Illustrations must be pasted in as soon as possible after the first mention of the illustration in the text, with the relevant caption underneath. This calls for some careful planning. If the illustration does not fill the page (20.3cm deep), leave a line space below the caption and then insert text in the remaining space.

Size of Illustrations

Illustrations may be inserted either "portrait" (maximum size 12.7cm wide by 20.3cm deep, including caption) or "landscape" (maximum size: 20.3cm wide by 12.7cm deep, including caption). Portrait illustrations are preferred. If necessary, extra-large figures may be divided and placed on two facing pages. Portrait figures may have text below them on the same page; landscape figures have no text on the same page, only the caption.

Preparation

Artwork must be of a high enough standard for direct reproduction; the publisher will not retouch it, and will reproduce it as it stands even if it is unsuitable, messy or illegible. Line drawings should be prepared in black (india) ink on white art paper or card, with all the lettering and symbols included. Computer-generated graphics of a similar high quality are also acceptable, as are good sharp photoprints ("glossies"). Computer print-outs must be completely legible. Axes of graphs should be properly labelled and appropriate units given.

Halftone Illustrations (photographs)

Good glossy original prints are required. Already printed photographs cut from other publications will not reproduce well (and usually will infringe copyright)! Have the halftone illustrations prepared so that they fit onto the page in either portrait or landscape format, or alternatively crop the illustration to the text width. Numbering, lettering and arrows may be inserted with rub-on letters.

Line Illustrations

The lettering on line illustrations must be satisfactory - not too large, not too small. The preferred style of lettering is "all capitals", with capital letters 2mm in height. It is usually easier to prepare line illustrations to a larger size (e.g. twice the required size), then have them reduced photographically for pasting into the text. In the reduced size the letters should be equal to or slightly smaller then letters in the main text. Authors are advised that improper preparation of lettering of figures is among the most common causes for delay in publications.

Figure Captions

After preparing each illustration, measure the depth of each (ignoring white borders, of course). Add 1.5cm (0.75") to the depth, and leave this amount of space in the text. Type the figure caption after the space has been measured on the page. Figures should be numbered with consecutive arabic numerals. In books, the figures are often numbered by chapters — e.g. Figure 1.1, 1.2, 2,1, etc (if the chapter number is not known, merely number figures 1, 2, 3, etc). Type Figure 1.1, etc. Leave three typewriter spaces, then type the caption like an ordinary sentence. If the caption is less than one line long, it should be centred under the figure. If it is more than one line long, it should be set over to the left-hand margin of the text and should be typed across the full width of the column, not the width of the figure. After the caption, leave one line of white space before starting the text.

Tables

All tables must be mentioned in the text and should appear as soon as possible after the first text reference. They may be set in a smaller typeface than the rest of the text if this is possible.

Numbering

Use arabic numerals according to chapter set in capitals (Table 1.1, 1.2, 2.1, etc). If the chapter number is not known, merely number tables 1, 2, 3, etc.

Captions

Type the caption at the head of the table, not the foot, set over to the left-hand margin of the table. Run on the table heading after three typewriter spaces, written like an ordinary sentence and ending with a full stop.

Planning

It may be necessary to type out a draft of some tables on a separate sheet of paper, to make sure that they fit. In any case, tables can be typed separately, then pasted in like illustrations. Tables should be centred in the text (see instructions for illustrations). If tables cannot conveniently be typed within the 12.7cm (5") width of the page, there are three other possibilities:

1. Type the table sideways on the page ("landscape")
2. Type the table to spread over two facing pages.
3. Type the table on a separate sheet, then have it reduced photographically to fit into the page. But remember that it must still be legible when reduced, as the pages are reduced again by 10% before printing.

Column Headings

Headings are usually ranged left over the columns, in italics if this typeface is available. Align the top lines of the headings with each other, to leave any space below (not above) shorter headings.

Data

Data should be arranged so that columns of like material read vertically, not horizontally, and should be ranged left in columns.

Rules

Draw horizontal rules (lines) on each table at the head of the table, at the foot, and after the column headings. These lines may be added with pen and ruler (using black ink) after the page has been typed. Do not add vertical lines to tables. Horizontal lines may also be added to indicate subheadings associated with a main heading.

Footnotes

These are designed by superior lower case letters (a, b, c, etc.) and should be typed below the table. Use footnotes for explaining abbreviations, symbols, data collecting methods, etc.

References And Notes

References are indicated in the text by the two alternative systems described below.

Harvard Style

References and notes are indicated in the text by the name and date system: either "Recent work (Cowan, 1984) ..." or "Recently Cowan (1984)...". If more than three authors are listed, cite the reference as "Cowan *et al.* (1984)...". However, in the end reference list, the first six authors should be given then "*et al.*" used. When citing more than one reference at a time, list them in chronological order, then in alphabetical order if there is more than one in the same year (e.g. "Smith, 1980; Fairclough 1981; Green, 1981"). If there is more than one publication by the same author(s) in the same year, distinguish by adding a, b, c, etc. to both the text citation and the list of references (e.g. "Smith, 1980a"). References should be collected and typed at the end of the paper in alphabetical order according to the first author.

Vancouver Style

References and notes are indicated in the text by consecutive superior arabic numerals (without parentheses). The full list should be collected and typed at the end of the paper in numerical order. On multiauthor references, all the authors' names should be listed up tot the first six, then "*et al.*" may be used.

Reference List

Type the reference list in single-line spacing. Listed references should be complete in all details, including article titles and journal titles in full. If italic typeface is not available, underline journal and book titles.

Journal article

Jordan, T.J., Grallo, R., Mashberg, D., Gordon, L. and Kapila, R. (1987) Manifestations of AIDS in intravenous drug users: a psychological approach. *Psychology and Health,* 1, 165–178.

Chapter in book

Gupta, R. (1987) Food for thought. *In Lattice Gauge Theory Using Parallel Processors*, edited by A. Zichichi, pp. 449–616. London: Gordon and Breach.

Book

Talley, W.K.(1967) *Transport Carrier Costing,* 2nd edn, pp. 35-39. London: Gordon and Breach.

Thesis

Griffiths, E. (1970) Sensory feedback in human posture control. *Sc*D *Thesis*, Centre for Movement Research, MIT, Boston, USA.

Proceedings

Carruthers, M. (1978) Ambulatory monitoring of air crew. *In Proceedings of the Second International Symposium on Ambulatory Monitoring* (Paris, 1977), edited by F.D. Scott, pp 23-27. London: Gordon and Breach.

Corporate author

British Ship Research Association (1976) *A Critical Evaluation of the Data on Wave Force Coefficients*, Report No. W278, 27 pp. London: BSRA

NB It is especially important to check that all the references cited in the text are included in the end list. Authors must check that reference details are correct and complete; otherwise the references are useless.

Scientific Terminology

Numbers

Set out as follows:

one to nine in words (but with units use numerals – 1 g, 5kHz, etc)

10, 100, 1000 (no comma), 10 000 (thin space, no comma)

1 000 0000 or one million *but* 1 million

$16 (not $16.00), $5.45

Decimals: 6.9 (point on the line), 0.78 (not .78), 1.5 (not 1.50), 20g (not 20.0g)

one-half, three-quarters (in text only)

20% (not "percent" in words, unless the number is also written in full at the beginning of a sentence)

When a sentence begins with a number, write it out in full (e.g. "Eighty-give percent"). If this is difficult, e.g. "Five men, 15 women and 12 children", try to rewrite the sentence.

Measurements and Units

Measurements and units are expressed with their proper abbreviations in metric SI units. The six basic SI units are:

Length: meter (m)	Time: second (s)
Mass: kilogram (kg)	Temperature: Celsius (°C)
Electric current: ampere (A)	Luminous intensity: candela (cd)

Note especially the following SI units and abbreviations:

Force: newton (N), not jg force
Work and energy of any kind: joule (J), not erg
Power of any kind: watt (W) Voltage: (v)
Light flux: lumen (lm)
Radioactivity: curie (Ci)

Note the abbreviations for minute (min), hour (h) and litre (l not L), and especially microgram (ug) and microlitre (ul). For cubic centimetres, use cm3 and for liquid measures ml (not cc or c.c.). There are no full stops or plurals when the official abbreviations are used. The prefixes k, m, u, n and p should be used where appropriate. It is preferable to avoid non-metric units, but if essential they may be used in parentheses after the proper SI unit. Measurements of blood pressure should be in mmHg.

INDEX

A

B

C

I

J

K

L

M

Q

R

V

W